# Headache

**Series Editor**
Paolo Martelletti, Roma, Italy

The purpose of this Series, endorsed by the European Headache Federation (EHF), is to describe in detail all aspects of headache disorders that are of importance in primary care and the hospital setting, including pathophysiology, diagnosis, management, comorbidities, and issues in particular patient groups. A key feature of the Series is its multidisciplinary approach, and it will have wide appeal to internists, rheumatologists, neurologists, pain doctors, general practitioners, primary care givers, and pediatricians. Readers will find that the Series assists not only in understanding, recognizing, and treating the primary headache disorders, but also in identifying the potentially dangerous underlying causes of secondary headache disorders and avoiding mismanagement and overuse of medications for acute headache, which are major risk factors for disease aggravation. Each volume is designed to meet the needs of both more experienced professionals and medical students, residents, and trainees.

Pınar Yalınay Dikmen • Aynur Özge
Editors

# Clinical Scales for Headache Disorders

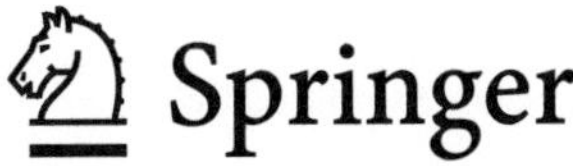 Springer

*Editors*
Pınar Yalınay Dikmen
Department of Neurology
Acıbadem University School of Medicine
İstanbul, Turkey

Aynur Özge
Department of Neurology
Mersin University Faculty of Medicine
Mersin, Turkey

ISSN 2197-652X        ISSN 2197-6538   (electronic)
Headache
ISBN 978-3-031-25940-1        ISBN 978-3-031-25938-8   (eBook)
https://doi.org/10.1007/978-3-031-25938-8



This Springer imprint is published by the registered company Springer Nature Switzerland AG
The registered company address is: Gewerbestrasse 11, 6330 Cham, Switzerland

# Foreword

In almost 30 years, headache medicine has moved from the descriptive, anecdotal phase, poor in classification criteria, clinical scales, and guidelines to a modern science, hinged on scientific evidence, diagnostic pathways and algorithms and targeted treatment plans, tools that serve as a solid guide in medical practice towards precise clinical definitions and the correct use of innovative and effective molecules.

Unfortunately, as the absence of diagnostic biomarkers that can be used in daily clinical practice in primary headaches persists, the use of clinical scales represents an indispensable refinement tool for both the clinical physician and the researcher.

This book summarizes in detail Clinical Scales and Patient Reported Outcome Measures in the domains of Diagnostic Screening, Impact and Burden, Quality of Life, Monitoring, Comorbidities, and miscellaneous.

The definition and accuracy of this series of questionnaires, which have been widely validated as clinical measurement tools, now lead us to consider them a cornerstone in clinical practice and an asset in a flourishing phase of continuous enhancement. These scales, which are already widely integrated in the design of randomized clinical trials and in the verification of the efficacy of treatments, should be integrated in the future operational revision of the International Classification of Headache Disorders, which would make it more clinically adherent.

The exponential growth of headache medicine, which is now rooted in the highest positions among the non-communicable social pathologies, has over the years obtained a solid basis of validation of the specificity and sensitivity of these clinical scales in area scientific journals, guaranteeing their support in accuracy and precision in diagnostic procedures.

This book aims to offer the physician and researcher a structured and agile compendium to support the clinical medicine of primary headaches and at the same time to facilitate its use as a ready-made reading list.

In presenting the 15th volume of the Headache Book Series, endorsed by the European Headache Federation, I want to confirm the continuity of seeding within the educational furrow dedicated to headache, and I wish it too to serve as a safe and lasting guide in clinical and research practice to ensure that individuals with headache have a proper level of Good Health and Wellbeing in line with United Nations Sustainable Development Goals 3.

Sapienza University                                              Paolo Martelletti
Rome, Italy

# Preface

Throughout human history, headache has been a common experience shared by people all over the world. Since the time of Hippocrates, physicians have attempted to transform the subjective symptoms of headaches into measurable, objective data. This book is devoted to this crucial and fundamental goal, concentrating on the clinical scales that are commonly employed in current headache studies as well as clinical practice. The book provides comprehensive theoretical information and covers the main areas of focus.

We begin by providing an overview of the current guidelines for headache and migraine medicine. In Chap. 2, we introduce readers to various clinical scales and Patient Reported Outcome Measures (PROMs). In Chap. 3, we provide detailed information on the reliability and validity of these instruments and move on to discuss individual questions or validated multi-item instruments. In Chap. 4, we offer a general framework for PROM development and evaluation. In Chap. 5, we delve into clinical scales and PROMs for measuring pain intensity. In Chap. 6, we discuss clinical scales and PROMs for diagnosing and screening headache and migraine. In Chap. 7, we give information about the instruments regarding assessing disability, impact, and burden of headache disorders. Chapter 8 provides a comprehensive discussion of PROMs for migraine and cluster headache, while Chap. 9 introduces readers to all scales related to psychiatric comorbidities frequently observed in headache disorders. Moving on to treatment monitoring and optimization, we present clinical instruments in Chap. 10 and highlight some unrecognized but useful clinical scales in headache studies in Chap. 11. Lastly, we dedicate Chap. 12 to clinical scales specifically used for children and adolescents. A summarized list of the current PROMs included in this book, categorized according to their scope, can be found in Fig. 1.

The book's chapters were authored by distinguished experts in the Headache Scientific Society, with several of them being the creators of currently used PROMs. We express our sincere gratitude to all authors who generously shared their invaluable knowledge and experience with us.

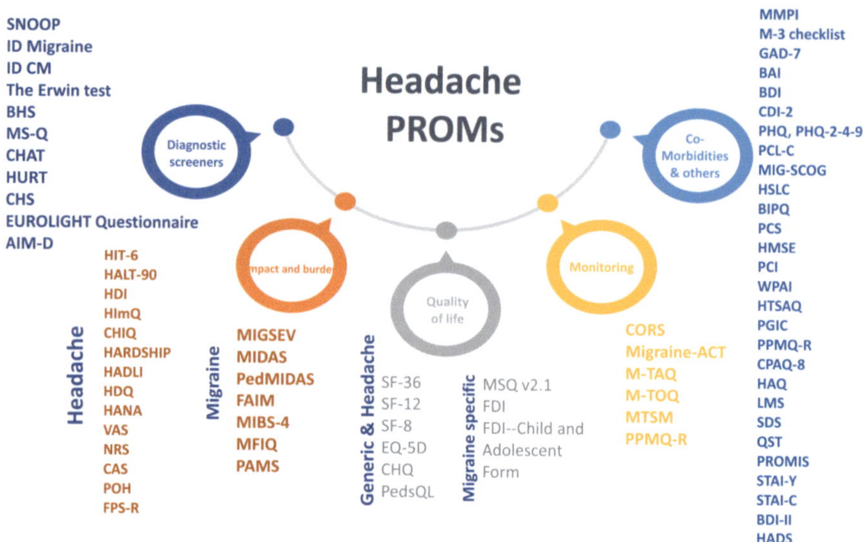


**Fig. 1** A summarized list of PROMs is given in this book for headache and migraine. PROM, Patient-reported outcome measure; CM, Chronic migraine; BHS, Brief Headache Screen; MS-Q, Migraine Screen Questionnaire; CHAT, The Computerized Headache Assessment Tool; HURT, The Headache Under-Response to Treatment; CHS, Cluster Headache Scale; AIM-D, The Activity Impairment in Migraine-Diary; HIT-6, Headache Impact Test-6; HALT-90, Headache-Attributed Lost Time Index; HDI, Henry Ford Headache Disability Inventory; HImQ, Headache Impact Questionnaire; CHIQ, Cluster Headache Impact Questionnaire; HARDSHIP, Headache-Attributed Restriction, Disability, Social Handicap and Impaired Participation Questionnaire; HADLI, Headache Activities of Daily Living Index; HDQ, Headache Disability Questionnaire; HANA, Headache Needs Assessment Survey; VAS, Visual Analogue Scale; NRS, Numeric Rating Scale; CAS, Coloured Analogue Scale; POH, Pieces of hurt tool; FPS-R, The Faces Pain Scale-Revised; MIGSEV, Migraine Severity Scale; MIDAS, Migraine Disability Assessment Questionnaire; PedMIDAS, Pediatric Migraine Disability Assessment; FAIM, Functional Assessment in Migraine Questionnaire; MIIBS-4, Migraine Interictal Burden Scale-4; MFIQ, Migraine Functional Impact Questionnaire; PAMS, The Pediatric and Adolescent Migraine Screen; SF-36, Short Form 36; SF-12, Short Form 12; SF-8, Short Form 8; ED-5Q, EuroQoL Quality of Life Scale; CHQ, Cluster Headache Quality of life scale; PedsQL, Pediatric Quality of Life Inventory; MSQ v2.1, Migraine Specific Quality of Life version 2.1; FDI, Functional Disability Inventory; CORS, Completeness of Response to migraine therapy; Migraine-ACT, Migraine Assessment of Current Therapy; M-TAQ, Migraine-Treatment Assessment Questionnaire; M-TOQ, Migraine-Treatment Optimization Questionnaire; MTSM, Migraine-Treatment Satisfaction Measure; PPMQ-R, Patient Perception of Migraine Questionnaire-Revised; MMPI, Minnesota Multiphasic Personality Inventory; M-3 Checklist, My Mood Monitor; GAD-7, Generalized Anxiety Disorder-7; BAI, Beck Anxiety Inventory; BDI, Beck Depression Inventory; CDI-2, Children's Depression Inventory 2; PHQ, Patients Health Questionnaire; PCL-C, PTSD Checklist-Civilian Version; MIG-SCog, Subjective Cognitive Impairments Scale; HSLC, Headache-Specific Locus of Control Scale; BIPQ, Brief Illness Perception Questionnaire; PCS, Pain Catastrophizing Scale; HMSE, Headache Management Self-Efficacy Scale; PCI, Pain-Coping Inventory; WPAI, Work Productivity and Activity Impairment Questionnaire; HTSAQ, The Headache Triggers Sensitivity and Avoidance Questionnaire; PGIC, Patient Global Impression Change Scale; PPMQ-R, Patient Perception of Migraine Questionnaire-Revised; CPAQ-8, Chronic Pain Acceptance Questionnaire; HAQ, The Headache Acceptance Questionnaire; LMS, The Loneliness of Migraine Scale; SDS, Severity of Dependence Scale; QST, Quantitative Sensory Testing; PROMIS, Patient-Reported Outcomes Measurement Information System; STAI-Y, The State-Trait Anxiety Inventory for older children; STAI-C, The State-Trait Anxiety Inventory for younger children; HADS, The Hospital Anxiety and Depression Scale

The production of this book would not have been possible without the invaluable support of the Springer team. The English edition was professionally executed to ensure ease of readability. However, it should be noted that the book does not aim to cover all PROM scales found in the literature in a chronological order. Our hope is that this book will prove beneficial to headache practitioners and researchers alike, ultimately leading to fewer painful days for headache patients.

Istanbul, Turkey<br>
Mersin, Turkey<br>
2022

Pınar Yalınay Dikmen<br>
Aynur Özge

# Acknowledgement

Editors thank Global Migraine and Pain Society for the language edition and secretarial support.

# Contents

# Chapter 1
# What Is the Best Methodology for Headache or Migraine Research?

Cristina Gaglianone, Enrico Bentivegna, and Paolo Martelletti

## 1.1 Introduction

Headache is a neurological disorder with a high disabling potential, characterised by painful episodes of moderate to severe intensity usually single-sided. Accompanying symptoms can be associated with the migraine episode which are often very characteristic and are represented by nausea, photophobia and phonophobia [1].

Migraine is a condition characterised by a high prevalence. In fact, it is estimated that the prevalence of migraine is 12% of the general population [2–4]. Migraine is about three times more prevalent in women than men. Indeed, the prevalence is around 6% for men, it rises to 16% for women. Furthermore, women usually have longer and more intense migraine attacks and experience a greater number of relapses resulting in a high level of disability [5].

Migraines have a significant effect on the quality of life of patients, especially when attacks become frequent. Not surprisingly, the Global Burden of Diseases, Injuries, and Risk Factors studies define migraine as one of the ten most disabling disorders in the world [6]. To date, headache represents the first neurological cause of disability, mainly under the age of 50.

An important aspect linked to this condition is represented by ictal and interictal burden to the patients and high economic costs to the society that it entails: on the one hand for the patient in terms of money spent on medical visits, therapies and examinations to which he/she undergoes, on the other in terms of reduced productivity. In fact, headache represents one of the first causes of absence from work with a percentage of about 20% of workdays lost every year [7, 8].

C. Gaglianone (✉) · E. Bentivegna · P. Martelletti
Department of Clinical and Molecular Medicine, Sapienza University, Rome, Italy

Regional Referral Headache Centre, Sant'Andrea Hospital, Rome, Italy
e-mail: cristina.gaglianone@uniroma1.it; enrico.bentivegna@uniroma1.it;
paolo.martelletti@uniroma1.it


P. Yalınay Dikmen, A. Özge (eds.), *Clinical Scales for Headache Disorders*,
Headache, https://doi.org/10.1007/978-3-031-25938-8_1

Despite the broad social impact of this condition, migraine frequently remains widely underdiagnosed and undertreated [2].

To overcome this problem, organisations and agencies such as the International Headache Society (IHS), the European Headache Federation (EHF), the Food and Drug Administration (FDA) and the European Medical Agency (EMA) conceived guidelines in order to help physicians to improve the management of migraine patient not merely for a correct diagnosis and for treatment of painful symptoms, but also all accompanying symptoms which represent a notable limitation in the patient's life. It is important that clinical practice always adheres to scientific evidence in order to ensure the best standard of care for patients.

Furthermore, the importance of knowledge of the guidelines is highlighted in the field of research. The quality of a clinical research fully dependent on adherence to guidelines: a strict adherence to guidelines represents a real tool for assessing the quality of a study and allows the comparison of the various clinical studies with each other [9].

This chapter will show current headache guidelines and try to provide guidance on how a headache research study should be conducted.

## Guidelines

In the field of headaches, guidelines represent a valuable tool to which physicians must refer in the management of the migraine patient in order to ensure the best standard of care for patients. Indeed, guidelines lead to the physician in every clinical decision, from diagnosis to therapy up to patient follow-up.

1. *First meeting with the migraine patient:*

    (a) *Classification*

The diagnosis of primary headache is substantially clinical and based on diagnostic criteria that refer to the International Classification of Headache Disorders (ICHD-3) [10]. Migraine has two main subtypes; migraine with aura and migraine without aura (Fig. 1.1).

*Migraine without aura:*
- *A: At least five attacks that meet criteria B and D:*
- *B:* Headache attacks lasting 4–72 h (when untreated or unsuccessfully treated)
- *C: Headache has at least two of the following characteristics:*

    - *Unilateral localization*
    - *Pulsating quality*
    - *Moderate or severe pain intensity*
    - Aggravation by or causing avoidance of routine physical activity

- *D:* During headache at least one of the following:

    - *Nausea and / or vomiting*
    - *Photophobia and / or phonophobia*

- *E:* Not better accounted for by another ICHD-3 diagnosis (Fig. 1.1).

| Migraine without aura | Migraine with aura | Chronic migraine |
| --- | --- | --- |
| **A.** At least 5 attacks that meet criteria **B** and **D**; | **A.** At least two attacks *that fulfil* criteria **B** and **C**; | Headache occurring on 15 or more days/ month for more than three months, which, on at least eight days/month, has the features of migraine headache. |
| **B.** Headache attacks lasting 4–72 hours (when untreated or unsuccessfully treated); | **B.** One or more of the following fully reversible aura symptoms:<br>1. *Visual;*<br>2. *Sensory;*<br>3. *speech and/or language;*<br>4. *Motor;*<br>5. *Brainstem;*<br>6. *Retinal.* | |
| **C.** Headache has at least 2 of the following characteristics:<br>- *Unilateral localization;*<br>- *Pulsating quality;*<br>- *Moderate or severe pain intensity;*<br>- *Aggravation by or causing avoidance of routine physical activity;* | **C.** At least three of the following six characteristics:<br>1. *At least one aura symptom spreads gradually in 5 or more minutes;*<br>2. *Two or more aura symptoms occur in succession;*<br>3. *Each individual aura symptom lasts 5–60 minutes;*<br>4. *At least one aura symptom is unilateral;*<br>5. *At least one aura symptom is positive:*<br>6. *The aura is accompanied, or followed within 60 minutes, by headache.* | |
| **D.** During headache at least one   of the following:<br>- *Nausea and / or vomiting;*<br>- *Photophobia and / or phonophobia.* | **D.** Not better accounted for by another ICHD-3 diagnosis. | |
| **E.** Not better accounted for by another ICHD-3 diagnosis | | |

**Fig. 1.1** Diagnostic criteria for headache according to the International Headache Society

It is possible that patients meet criteria for "migraine without aura" but have fewer than five attacks. In that case, they should be coded as "probable migraine without aura". The patient falls asleep with a headache but wakes up without it, the moment of awakening is calculated as the end of the migraine attack.

Frequently, migraine attacks can be preceded by prodromal symptoms. These can begin hours or even days before pain comes off. These are fatigue, difficulty concentrating, sensitivity to light and/or sound, stiffness of the neck muscles, nausea, blurred vision. Postdrome symptoms may also be associated with the migraine attack. The most frequent ones are fatigue and difficulty concentrating.

It is worth noting that in a minority of women (about 10%) migraine attacks occur in association with the menstrual cycle. Most of these attacks take the form of migraine attacks without aura and can be classified as follows:

- *Pure menstrual migraine without aura:* Occurs exclusively on days −2 to +3 of menstruation in at least two out of three menstrual periods and at no other stage of the cycle.

- *Menstrually related migraine without aura:* Attacks occur on days −2 to +3 of menstruation on at least two out of three menstrual cycles and on other days of the cycle.
- *Non-menstrual migraine without aura:* Migraine attacks are unrelated to menstruation.

Attacks that occur in conjunction with the menstrual period tend to be particularly intense and disabling, lasting longer and combined with more intense nausea than attacks occurring beyond the menstrual period [11].

Migraine shows peculiar features during the developmental age; in fact, migraine is more often bilateral in children and adolescents, while unilateral pain usually emerges in late adolescence or early adult life. The duration of the attacks varies between 1 and 72 h. Pain usually has frontotemporal localization while occipital pain is rarer and must be carefully evaluated. The presence of photophobia or phonophobia must be deduced from the child's behaviour during the migraine attack.

It is possible to identify periodic childhood syndromes as possible precursors of migraine. These are represented by:

- Cyclic vomiting syndrome: Patients suffer from an episodic nausea and vomiting characterised by recurrent stereotypic symptoms with disease-free intervals.
- Abdominal migraine: Recurrent idiopathic abdominal pain disorder of varying duration, moderate or severe intensity and associated with symptoms such as nausea and vomiting. Again, the patient is asymptomatic during the intercritical periods.
- Benign paroxysmal vertigo: These symptoms occur in completely healthy children in the form of repeated and brief dizziness which resolves spontaneously [11].

**Migraine with aura:**
This condition is characterised by recurrent attacks, lasting minutes, of unilateral transient and fully reversible visual, sensory, or other central nervous system symptoms that usually develop gradually and are usually followed by headache and associated migraine symptoms.

The diagnostic criteria are:

- A. At least two attacks *that fulfil* criteria B and C
- B. One or more of the following fully reversible aura symptoms:

  - visual
  - sensory
  - speech and/or language
  - motor
  - brainstem
  - retinal

- C. At least three of the following characteristics:

  - at least one aura symptom spreads gradually in 5 or more minutes
  - two or more aura symptoms occur in succession

  – each individual aura symptom lasts 5–60 min
  – at least one aura symptom is unilateral
  – at least one aura symptom is positive
  – the aura is accompanied, or followed within 60 min, by headache

- D. Not better accounted for by another ICHD-3 diagnosis (Fig. 1.1).

Approximately 1% of patients with migraine experience both migraine episodes with aura and without aura; in these patients both forms of headache must be diagnosed and subsequently coded.

The visual aura is the most common type of aura and affects about 90% of patients, followed by sensory disturbances. If multiple aura symptoms are present, they tend to occur in succession. Commonly, visual symptoms are the first to appear. When the aura is accompanied by motor weakness, the disorder is classified as "hemiplegic migraine".

It is always important to take care of the presence of the aura without headache for which a careful evaluation is certainly necessary in order to diagnose the presence of a secondary form of headache and a possible underlying pathology such as a transient ischemic attack. In particular, if the onset of the aura is after age 40 or if negative symptoms prevail, if the duration of the aura is >60 min or if it develops very rapidly (<5 min), it should be necessary to resort to further investigations in order to make a correct diagnosis. When these features are present or in case of concomitant cerebrovascular diseases, experts recommend performing CT angiography or MRI of the carotid and vertebral arteries [12, 13].

**Frequency of Migraine**
Based on a patient' headache frequency, migraine has two subtypes; episodic and chronic migraine. Episodic migraine is characterised by those with migraine who have zero to 14 headache days per month. Chronic migraine is defined as a headache occurring on 15 or more days/month for more than 3 months, of which 8 days/month or more days meet criteria for migraine without aura (Fig. 1.1).

For a correct diagnosis of chronic migraine, headache diaries are generally used in which patients can record information on pain, associated symptoms and therapy every day for at least 1 month.

Should not be underestimated that the main cause of chronic headache is drug abuse. In this case, the diagnosis of "medication overuse headache" must be added to the diagnosis of chronic migraine. About 50% of patients who resort to drug abuse return to an episodic type of migraine after discontinuation [10].

(b) *Diagnosis*

The diagnosis of migraine is essentially clinical and is based on two fundamental items as follows an anamnesis and a physical examination.

Careful collection of anamnestic data is essential in the diagnosis of migraine. Thus headache can be classified according to the ICHD-3 criteria and a physician can collect all useful information to exclude any other secondary pathologies [2].

The history should be followed by a careful physical examination, both general and neurological [2].

In order to make a diagnosis of primary headache, neither the history nor the physical examination should suggest a secondary cause for headache. Once a secondary cause for headache has been excluded, no further investigations are usually required [14].

The history has to focus on:

– Age of headache onset;
– Pain characteristics (duration, intensity, frequency of attacks, localization);
– Accompanying symptoms (nausea, vomiting, photophobia, phonophobia, osmophobia but also possible lacrimation, conjunctival injection, rhinorrhea, etc.);
– Family history of migraine;
– Triggering or precipitating factors (stress, cough, neck movements, intake of particular foods) or relationship between migraine and menstrual cycle;
– Consequences of headache on daily activities;
– Drugs taken for a headache;
– Coexisting conditions and comorbidities (insomnia, depression, anxiety, hypertension, asthma and history of heart disease or stroke) [15].

The physical examination must focus on:

– General physical examination which includes measurement of blood pressure and heart rate;
– Neurological examination (general evaluation of mental status, examination of cranial nerves and eye movements, evaluation of facial movements and their symmetry, evaluation of limb strength, reflexes, gait evaluation, etc.);
– Neck exam (posture, movement and palpation for muscle pain points)
– Examination of the paranasal sinuses, carotid arteries as well as temporomandibular joints;
– Specific tests if, following the physical examination, the clinician deems them necessary or as an aid to the correct diagnosis [15].

Headache is certainly well represented by the *clinical diary* on which the patient can write down all the information relating to the migraine episode and which the clinician can use not only to make an initial diagnosis; but also, if necessary, for its possible subsequent re-evaluation.

### (c) *When to suspect a secondary condition*

Although headache is caused by a primary headache disorder for many cases, it is important to emphasise that several neurological diseases, often very serious, may mimic a benign headache disorder.

If the physician is not sure about the primary nature of the headache, the patient should undergo additional investigations which are not usually required in normal clinical practice.

Indicators of a possible secondary form of headache can be:

- Thunderclap headache onset, fever and meningism, papilledema with focal signs or reduced level of consciousness, etc. These conditions can represent real neurological emergencies;
- Severe systemic disease;
- Focal neurological signs, atypical headaches, elderly patients with cognitive change or headache onset after 50 years of age, worsening of pain following neck movements or pain following physical exertion [15].

Unless the patient manifests neurological signs and symptoms, it is possible to resort to second level tests such as MRI, MR angiography or CT.

### (d) *Therapy*

Before starting therapy for migraine, it would be advisable to have an interview with the patient for explaining all possible benefits and side effects of acute and preventive treatments. Indeed, a purpose of preventive treatment is not to cure migraine but it is possible to achieve satisfactory results in reducing the frequency and intensity of migraine attacks. The interview with the patient attempts to identify, if present, any triggering factors and, when possible, eliminate them (promoting, for example, a correct lifestyle). Although a relatively large amount of migraine medications are available today, only about 50% of patients get satisfactory responses from therapy [16]. This is probably related to a series of genetic variants of the patient that influence the pharmacokinetics and pharmacodynamics [17].

Regarding migraine therapy, we can refer to acute therapies and preventive treatments. In order to choose the best treatment for our patient, we must take into account several aspects: both the efficacy of a drug and its tolerability, the contraindications that the patient may present, as well as the availability of that therapy. The patient could access many innovative drugs only in specialised centres, for example. Another important issue is the degree of disability that the headache involves in the patient's life. The approach to migraine therapy must take place step by step (stepped management) by treating at least three consecutive migraine attacks with the same therapy before switching to another drug [18].

Among the therapies for acute migraine attacks, two classes of drugs are mainly available [18]:

- Non-specific drugs for migraine: These are mainly non-opioid analgesics, basically represented by nonsteroidal anti-inflammatory drugs (NSAIDs). Among the most effective, we find ibuprofen (also used in the paediatric population), N-acetyl salicylic acid and diclofenac. These are over-the-counter drugs that the patient has free access to and are widely used. Although they represent a good therapeutic choice in sporadic cases of headache, their use in chronic cases is not recommended due to their possible side effects mainly related to their gastric injury.

  Paracetamol is a drug that can be used in case of allergies or contraindications to NSAIDs (e.g. gastrointestinal bleeding or pregnancy), however this has proved to be of little effect in the treatment of migraine.

Since migraine attacks are often associated with accompanying symptoms such as nausea and vomiting, it may be useful to resort to drugs for treating these symptoms. The most used for this purpose are prokinetics and antiemetics, represented mainly by domperidone and metoclopramide.

Drugs such as opioids and barbiturates should be avoided which are accompanied by many side effects and can be addictive, in addition to being ineffective for migraine (Fig. 1.2).

– Specific drugs: The most used are Triptans. This class of drugs represented a real breakthrough in headache therapy. These are effective and well tolerated drugs in most migraine patients and in case of failure of a particular molecule it is possible to obtain a therapeutic response with a different molecule. Triptans have proven to be particularly effective if taken in the initial stages of the attack, when the pain is still mild, while it is not yet clear whether they act on the symptoms of the aura. Most triptans are taken orally. However, sumatriptan can be taken by subcutaneous injection and zolmitriptan as a nasal spray, thus offering a great advantage in case the patient experiences nausea or vomiting.

Triptans are contraindicated in pregnancy, in uncontrolled arterial hypertension and in patients with cardiovascular and cerebrovascular diseases, and should be administered with caution in elderly patients.

If triptans were contraindicated or in case of their therapeutic failure (understood as inadequate or failed response to therapy in at least three consecutive migraine attacks), it is possible to employ other new classes of drugs such as Gepants and Ditans.

To date, the use of Ergotamine is not recommended due to poor efficacy and numerous side effects (Fig. 1.2).

| **Migraine Therapy** |
|---|
| **A.** Acute therapy: |
| - *Non-specific drugs for migraine: ibuprofen, N-acetyl salicylic acid, diclofenac, Paracetamol* |
| - *Specific drugs: Triptans, Gepants and Ditans* |
| - *Therapy for accompanying symptoms: Domperidone, metoclopramide* |
| **B.** Preventive therapy: |
| - *B blockers* |
| - *Amitriptyline* |
| - *Topiramate* |
| - *Candesartan* |
| - *Sodium valproate* |
| - *Flunarizine* |
| - *Monoclonal antibodies for CGRP* |
| - *Botulinum toxin A* |

**Fig. 1.2** Drugs that are used for acute, preventive treatments of migraine

A proper migraine therapy management is schematically summarised in Box 1.1.

> **Box 1.1 Management of Migraine Therapy**
>
> *Management of migraine therapy*
>
> - *Resort to acute therapy if the patient does not exceed two attacks per week;*
> - *Resort to preventive therapy in patients with frequent attacks or when these seriously compromise the quality of life despite adequate acute treatment;*
> - *Start with the lowest dose and possibly increase later in the absence of side effects;*
> - *Continue the therapy for at least 2/3 months before considering it ineffective;*
> - *When choosing the drug, evaluate its availability on the market which varies in different countries;*
> - *Inform the patient that excessive and inappropriate use of drugs can cause chronic headaches;*
> - *Evaluate the patient's adherence to prophylactic therapy, if necessary, resort to the use of clinical diaries*

The drugs that can be used for preventive treatment of migraine [18]:

- B blockers;
- Amitriptyline;
- Topiramate;
- Candesartan;
- Sodium valproate;
- Flunarizine;
- Monoclonal antibodies for CGRP;
- Botulinum toxin A (Fig. 1.2).

Recently, several compounds aimed at interfering with the CGRP signalling pathway are introduced in commerce [19, 20]. Gepants, with the advantage of the oral administration [21–23], appear to provide good results. Other therapeutic strategies and new drugs directed against other signalling pathways of the trigeminothalamic system have been developed: molecules targeting glutamate, PACAP, orexin or ion channels are showing encouraging results. Considering this proliferation of several effective therapeutic options, a guide to understanding the approach for each patient management becomes essential. Much remains to be studied about the pathophysiological underlying this complex disease to refine the therapeutic targets and the development of correct strategies for migraine management. To this end, we take the liberty of speculating that personalised medicine could help us to define more precisely the most effective molecule for the individual patient [24].

**Clinical Trial**

Planning a high quality clinical trial is a key step in advancing scientific research on a disease. In 1991, IHS was first developed and published guidelines for conducting controlled trials of migraine drugs [25]. Over the years, these guidelines have been modified and updated in accordance with the continuous innovations in the field of research and treatment for headache, reaching the current fourth edition.

The continuous updating of the guidelines aims to provide a standardised and evidence-based approach for the execution of randomised controlled trials for the treatment of migraine, to improve the results of these studies and to make them comparable to each other.

The standardisation of these studies represents a real tool for verifying the quality of a clinical study. A quality that is strictly dependent on the degree of adherence to the guidelines.

Clinical trials guidelines are an extremely important tool to ensure not only the uniformity and quality of clinical trials, but also the subsequent phases such as the identification of increasingly effective drugs and their commercialization, the management of patients with ability to guarantee the best standards of care, and so forth.

Despite the support they offer, adherence to guidelines has always remained low over the years (31% in the studies conducted between 2002 and 2008) [6] and this compromises not only the validity and quality of the study in question but also the possibility of comparing the data obtained.

The purpose of this chapter is to summarise and provide a simple guide for the publication of new clinical trials in the field of migraine.

In particular, we will try to guide the reader in conducting a clinical trial that may cover both acute and preventive treatment of episodic and chronic migraine separately for greater facilitation.

### Guidelines for Controlled Trials of Acute Treatment of Migraine Attacks

1. **Patient selection:** *Patients who can take part in the clinical trial must meet the diagnostic criteria for migraine according to the most updated version of the ICHD-3 according to the IHS.*

**Note:**
(a) Patients with secondary headache and patients diagnosed with MOH should be excluded from the study;
(b) Patients should have between 2 and 8 migraine attacks per month and at least 48 h must pass between two successive attacks. This time allows for better identification of the single migraine attack and avoids the use of multiple therapies during a single attack;
(c) Subjects must have fewer than 15 migraine attacks per month (thus, patients with chronic headache should be excluded in the acute therapy investigation phase);
(d) Headache must have been present for at least 1 year prior to inclusion in the clinical study and must have onset in the patient before age 50; indeed, as previously mentioned, the onset of this condition after the age of 50 is rare and should lead to suspicion of a secondary condition;
(e) Subjects must be between 18 and 65 years old, while subjects over the age of 65 can be included in post-marketing studies;
(f) Both male and female can be enrolled with the exclusion of pregnant or lactating women. For women of childbearing age it is necessary that the latter follow careful anti-contraceptive therapy.

(g) In studies where participants take therapies other than for migraine alone, the use of permitted medications should be pre-specified;

(h) Preventive treatment of migraine should be discontinued unless under study. This must be suspended at least 1 month before the start of the trial;

(i) Those who have taken antipsychotic and antidepressant therapy within the previous 3 months should be excluded.

2. **Trial design**: *The study of drugs intended for the acute treatment of migraine attacks should be conducted in randomised, double-blind, placebo-controlled trials.*

**Note:**

(a) Even when two active treatments are evaluated, a placebo control should be included to increase the sensitivity of the test;

(b) Randomization is essential to avoid bias and, in large studies, helps to homogenise groups;

(c) Both parallel and cross group projects can be used, however, the latter are often preferable for simplicity;

(d) Stratification is not usually required in acute therapy studies, but this can be considered when the two groups are not homogeneous or in the presence of a factor that could influence the results. In controlled migraine studies, the use of prognostic factor stratification should be limited to the only variables that, in previous studies, have been shown to influence the primary efficacy endpoint. Stratification variables include age, body weight, baseline, etc. Obviously, since migraine is a disease that primarily affects women, sex can be used as a stratification factor to control population imbalances.

(e) Effective doses of a standard drug should be used in comparative clinical studies using the known optimal therapeutic dose of the comparator (unless this is clinically inadequate);

(f) When available preclinical data show good pharmacokinetics (i.e. good bio-availability and rapid oral absorption) oral administration of the test treatment is recommended as this is the preferred route of administration in most patients with migraine [26]. Other routes of administration may be considered in particular conditions such as severe nausea;

(g) Timing of treatment during a migraine attack must be pre-established: participants need to receive clear instructions on when to resort to treatment; they must also be asked to record in the clinical diary the time and intensity of pain when taking the drug;

(h) The use of additional medications should be permitted in the event of failure of the treatment under consideration, but this should only occur after the time established as the efficacy endpoint has elapsed. If the intake occurs before the established time, it must be considered as a therapeutic failure of the drug in question;

(i) The response to treatment should be evaluated on at least four migraine attacks, one of which should be randomly treated with placebo;

(j) Assessment of tolerance to treatment should be based on long-term studies;

3. **Evaluation of the results and statistical analyses:** *Electronic or paper diaries should be used, in which patients should report predefined endpoints.*

Patients should report in their clinical diaries:

(a) the characteristics of the migraine attack;
(b) the presence of accompanying symptoms (such as nausea, vomiting, photophobia, phonophobia);
(c) timing of treatment (in particular, the time between the onset of painful symptoms and the taking of therapy);
(d) any adverse events that occur following treatment (particularly, if serious, they should be reported within 24 h of their onset).

As regards the statistical analysis, it is necessary to establish a priori various aspects including primary measurement time, primary efficacy endpoint, data collection methods, sample size, methods of comparison between the populations of subjects, the methods that will be used for the statistical analysis.

It is possible to use statistical software for the execution of tests and graphs and summary tables. To obtain satisfactory results, it is preferable to work on large samples and multi-centred trials.

4. **Endpoint:** *Primary and secondary endpoints must be clearly defined in a clinical trial.*

**Note:**
(a) A clinical trial can be considered effective if it reaches a predefined endpoint. Therefore, it is required that they are clearly established at the start of the trial;
(b) The endpoints used in the trial must follow a hierarchy and must be categorized into primary and secondary endpoints.
(c) **Primary endpoint:**

  - Pain freedom at 2 h: intended as the percentage of subjects who are pain free 2 h after the study therapy;

This endpoint was introduced only in the most recent versions of the IHS guidelines, replacing the endpoint of "headache relief" due to the high placebo response in migraine patients. The placebo effect is a phenomenon capable of widely influencing the results of clinical trials in various disease states. This is especially true in migraine treatment studies. Indeed, it has been seen that the response to placebo in headache relief can reach over 30%, while the response to placebo for the absence of pain is just about 9% [27, 28];

  - Freedom from the most bothersome symptom at 2 h;

(d) **Co-primary endpoint:**

  - Absence of the most disabling symptom 2 h after taking the therapy;

(e) **Secondary endpoints:**

- *Relapse:* New migraine attacks before 48 h have elapsed from the administration of the experimental treatment, in subjects with resolution of the painful symptoms within 2 h of taking the therapy.
- *Sustained pain freedom:* Defined as the percentage of asymptomatic patients 2 h after administration of therapy, with no use of additional therapy and who do not relapse 24 or 48 h after treatment;
- *Total freedom from migraine:* Defined as the absence of accompanying symptoms typical of migraine (among which the most typical are nausea, vomiting, photophobia and phonophobia) 2 h after treatment;
- *Headache intensity:* The intensity of the pain must be recorded in the clinical diary prior to taking pharmacological treatment, and subsequently assessed at predetermined times. According to the guidelines, it should be reassessed every 30 min up to 2 h after treatment, then every hour up to 4 h later, at 12, 24 and 48 h after treatment and at the time of relapse. It is possible to resort to the use of four-point scales where 0 indicates absence of pain and 4 indicates severe pain. Alternatively, a 100 mm visual analog scale (VAS) or ten-point numerical rating scale (NRS) can be used;
- *Time to pain freedom:* Assess the speed of response to therapy;
- *Rescue medication:* The percentage of patients using rescue medication within 2 h of trial treatment can be considered an indirect measure of effectiveness. As previously stated, this should be regarded as a therapeutic failure;
- *Global evaluation:* Takes into consideration the subject's point of view mainly on tolerability to therapy, particularly in phase II and III studies, as well as in studies comparing two or more active drugs;
- *Global impact:* This refers to the impact that the headache and accompanying symptoms have on the patient's quality of life. Functional disability and health-related quality of life are important secondary endpoints that have assumed an increasingly important role in acute therapy efficacy studies. For this purpose, a simple numerical scale from 0 to 4 can be used where 0 is no disability and 4 represents the maximum disability (inability to carry out normal daily actions or need for bed rest). Improving the quality of life is one of the main goals of migraine treatment;
- *Associated symptoms:* Since symptoms such as nausea, vomiting, photophobia and phonophobia are often present during a migraine attack, their resolution can represent a tool for evaluating the effectiveness of the therapy. Their presence should be recorded in the patient's diary at the time of administration of the treatment and at the time of the evaluation of the primary efficacy outcome (e.g. 2 h). However, it should be considered that symptoms such as nausea and vomiting may also represent an adverse treatment event;
- *Treatment preference:* It is a subjective evaluation in which both patient preferences and tolerance to therapy are taken into consideration;

- *Treatment of relapse:* Measured as the percentage of subjects with freedom from pain 2 h after administration of treatment for headache recurrence;
- *Adverse events*: The patient must note in his clinical diary any adverse events that occur during participation in the clinical trials, indicating their characteristics (e.g. pain intensity, onset and duration) as recommended by the International Conference on Harmonization's Guideline for good clinical practice [29]. Upon the occurrence of an adverse event, it is necessary to assess whether this was really determined by the treatment in question.

**Special Populations**

– **Patients with migraine attacks both with and without aura:** Because acute treatment studies can be conducted in populations of subjects who have only one type of migraine or both (with and without aura), researchers are unable to determine whether both types of migraine attacks have similar or different responses to treatment unless each attack is separately classified as migraine with aura or migraine without aura. Therefore, a detailed record of the characteristics of the aura is mandatory.

  The test protocol should clearly state whether the goal is to stop or minimise the duration of the aura or reduce or eliminate the headache, as these are distinct outcomes that most likely have different biological basis.
– **Children and adolescents:** Migraine attacks are generally short-lived in children and adolescents, and the placebo response tends to be high. The IHS is developing a separate set of recommendations for clinical trials on the acute and preventive treatment of migraine attacks in children and adolescents.

**Publication of Studies**

– The publication of the study results should include all primary and secondary endpoints and all safety data. Before starting any trial-related activities, a Steering Committee should agree on the timing for publication and, if possible, include them in the protocol; a Publication Committee may also be set up. At the end of the recruitment or at the beginning of the trial, a design paper with the reference data can be published. The authorship of the publications relating to the studies should be based on the criteria of the International Committee of Medical Journal Editors [30].
– The authors must declare the presence of conflicts of interest. Note that conflicts of interest extend to an investigator's close relatives (partner and children).
– The IHS recommends post-approval product registries (prospective observational studies) to evaluate the use of newly approved treatments in clinical practice. The logs generate real data on efficacy, tolerability and long-term safety. These registries may also include individuals with relevant comorbidities who were excluded from clinical trials for acute migraine.

**Guidelines for Controlled Trials of Preventive Treatment of Migraine Attacks in Episodic Migraine**

1. **Patient selection:** *Patients to be enrolled are those who meet the criteria for episodic migraine according to the current version of the ICHD (International Classification of Headache Disorders)* [31].

**Note:**

(a) Patients with headache with aura, headache without aura, tension-type headache or episodic attacks of other forms of primary headache can enter the trial while those with chronic headache should be excluded (i.e. subjects presenting more than 15 headache attacks per month);

(b) Episodic attacks of headache must have been present for at least 1 year before inclusion in the trial;

(c) The eligible subjects must be between 18 and 50 years old;

(d) Both men and women can be enrolled: pregnant or lactating women should be excluded while women of childbearing age should use appropriate prophylactic measures due to the possible teratogenic effects of the drug under investigation. Since migraine is present in the general population with a woman: man ratio of 3:1 it would be advisable, when possible, to respect this ratio in order to best represent real life;

(e) The trial should be divided into four main phases:

   - screening phase: this phase should have a duration of at least 4 weeks during which the eligibility criteria of the subjects are evaluated;
   - baseline: period of at least 4 months between the screening phase and the enrolment of patients in the trial; at this stage, patients should begin recording information about their migraine episodes in electronic journals in order to exclude patients with chronic headache or medication overuse;
   - double-blind period;
   - open-label period;

(f) If concomitant preventive treatments are allowed, they should belong to pharmaceutical classes different from the drug in question; furthermore, patients who resort to additional medications should undergo a stratified randomization so that the two groups are balanced;

(g) Subjects must record in electronic or paper diaries information regarding the characteristics of the headache (onset, accompanying symptoms, acute therapy used, time to disappearance of symptoms and any adverse events (AEs) to the drug; when AEs are serious these should be communicated within 24 h of their appearance).

2. **Trial design:** *a double-blind, randomized study should be conducted and the treatment under investigation compared with placebo* [31].

**Note:**

(a) Even when two active drugs are compared, a placebo control is recommended;

(b) Projects in parallel groups should be preferred;

(c) The double-blind treatment phase should last at least 24 weeks. Longer phases (for example 28 weeks) or open-label phases could be useful in order to evaluate the safety and tolerability of the treatment;

(d) In Phase 2 trial a broad spectrum of dosages can be tested while in Phase 3 one or two are tested;

3. **Endpoint:** *Primary and secondary endpoints need to be prospectively defined* [31].

(a) **Primary endpoint:**

- Change from baseline in migraine days per unit time;
- Change from baseline in moderate/severe headache days.

(b) **Secondary endpoint:**

- Reduction in migraine attacks;
- Onset of the effect of preventive treatment;
- Effect on the most disabling symptom

4. **Statistic:** *Analytic issues need to be prospectively defined; s*tatistical analysis must be based on methods and tests suitable for evaluating them.

**Guidelines for Controlled Trials of Preventive Treatment of Chronic Migraine**

1. **Patient selection:** *Patients to be enrolled are those who meet the criteria for chronic migraine according to the current version of the ICHD (International Classification of Headache Disorders)* [32].

**Note:**

(a) Patients with medication overuse headache can be enrolled but a stratified randomization of the two groups must be carried out so that the two groups are balanced; however, patients who overuse analgesics containing opioids or barbiturates or for those whose overuse of drugs has caused pathological consequences (e.g. peptic ulcer in patients who abuse NSAIDs) should be excluded;

(b) Headache must have been present for 15 or more days per month for at least 12 months prior to trial enrolment;

(c) Individuals with other types of primary headache may be admitted;

(d) Individuals over 18 years of age can be admitted. Headache episodes must have appeared before age 50 and chronic headache started before age 65;

(e) Both men and women can be admitted, however it would be preferable to respect the real man-woman ratio in the general population;

(f) Children or adolescents and subjects with secondary forms of headache must be excluded;

(g) Monotherapy studies are the best option to evaluate the efficacy and safety of a treatment. However, concomitant preventive therapy may be permitted as long as it has been taken for at least 3 months prior to the start of the trial and its intake remains constant and does not change during the trial;

2. **Trial design:** *Trials of preventive treatment of chronic migraine should be conducted in randomised, double-blind, placebo-controlled trials. It is preferable to use parallel groups and a stratified design* [32].

(a) Trial initiation must follow a baseline period of at least 28 days. This period is intended to verify that the subjects enrolled really meet the eligibility criteria of the trial. To this end, it is important that relevant information (for example the frequency of migraine attacks, their characteristics and the therapies taken) are recorded in clinical diaries;

(b) The duration of the trial must be at least 12 weeks, but longer periods are acceptable in order to obtain additional information in terms of efficacy, tolerability and safety.

3. **Endpoint:** *Primary and secondary endpoints need to be prospectively defined* [32].

(a) **Primary endpoint:**

- Change in migraine days;
- Change in moderate to severe headache days;
- Responder rate

The two endpoints that are not adopted as the primary endpoint should be selected as secondary ones.

(b) **Secondary endpoint** (in addition to the two endpoints mentioned above):

- Responder rate;
- Switch into episodic migraine;
- Switch medication overuse into non-medication overuse.
- Acute therapy;
- Quality of life, impact of headache on daily life or headache-related disability.

4. **Statistical analysis and publication of results:** *All statistical tools used for data analysis must be established a priori* [32].

(a) The planning of the statistical analysis must concern: the method of data collection, sample size, methodology of comparison of the two parallel groups, statistical analysis plan, imputation of missing data, etc.

(b) All results to which the research has led (both primary and secondary endpoints and safety data), both positive and negative, must be published in manuscript form.

Similarities and differences between trials that have been reported in this chapter have been summarized in Box 1.2.

**Box 1.2 Similarities and Differences Between Trials for Acute Therapy, Preventive Therapy for Episodic Headache and Chronic Headache**

**Patient selection**
Subjects who meet the diagnostic criteria of the recent version of the International Classification of Headache Disorders can be enrolled

| | |
|---|---|
| **Trials of acute treatment of migraine attacks** | *Inclusion criteria: 2–8 headache attacks per month, for at least a year prior, headache occurring before the age of 50.* |
| | *Exclusion criteria: secondary headache, chronic headache, or medication overuse* |
| **Trials of preventive treatment of migraine attacks in episodic migraine** | *Inclusion criteria: primary episodic headache for at least a year prior* |
| | *Exclusion criteria: chronic headache* |
| **Trials of preventive treatment of chronic migraine** | *Inclusion criteria: Headache present for ≤15 per month for at least 12 months prior, headache onset before age 50 and chronic before age 65* |
| | *Exclusion criteria: Secondary forms of headache* |

Trial design

| | |
|---|---|
| **Trials of acute treatment of migraine attacks** | *Randomised, double-blind, placebo-controlled trials* |
| **Trials of preventive treatment of migraine attacks in episodic migraine** | *Randomised, double-blind, placebo-controlled trials* |
| **Trials of preventive treatment of chronic migraine** | *Randomised, double-blind, placebo-controlled trials* |

Endpoint

| | |
|---|---|
| **Trials of acute treatment of migraine attacks** | *Primary endpoint: pain freedom at 2 h, freedom from the most bothersome symptom at hours, absence of the most disabling symptom 2 h after therapy* |
| | *Secondary endpoint: relapse, sustained pain freedom, total freedom from migraine, headache intensity, time to pain freedom, rescue medication, global evaluation, global impact, associated symptoms, treatment preference, treatment of relapse, adverse events* |
| **Trails of preventive treatment of migraine attacks in episodic migraine** | *Primary endpoint: change from baseline in migraine days per unit time; change from baseline in moderate/ severe headache days* |
| | *Secondary endpoint: reduction in migraine attacks, onset of the effect of preventive treatment, effect on the most disabling symptom* |
| **Trials of preventive treatment of chronic migraine** | *Primary endpoint: change in migraine days, change in moderate to severe headache days, responder rate* |
| | *Secondary endpoint: responder rate, switch into episodic migraine, switch medication overuse into non-medication overuse, acute therapy, quality of life, impact of headache on daily life or headache-related disability* |

## 1.2   Conclusions

Care of migraine patient always represented a great hurdle in the employment of the scientific field. This because, despite all the innovations and discoveries that have been made in recent years, the treatment of this pathology remains articulated and complex. Despite this, however, there are tools that are useful to who is faced with this pathology. These are represented by two fundamental elements which are evidence-based medicine and the guidelines that lead to therapeutic choices, and which ensure the best possible therapy. We hope that with this chapter we have been able to outline the path of the best research in the field of headache and that this can be useful in the management of this invalidating pathology.

**Acknowledgments**   n/a

**Funding**   This paper was not funded.

**Declaration of Interest**   The authors have no relevant affiliations or financial involvement with any organization or entity with a financial interest in or conflict with the subject matter or materials discussed in this manuscript.

# References

1. Pescador Ruschel MA, De Jesus O. Migraine headache. StatPearls Publishing; 2022.
2. Eigenbrodt AK, Ashina H, Khan S, Diener HC, Mitsikostas DD, Sinclair AJ, Pozo-Rosich P, Martelletti P, Ducros A, Lantéri-Minet M, Braschinsky M, Del Rio MS, Daniel O, Özge A, Mammadbayli A, Arons M, Skorobogatykh K, Romanenko V, Terwindt GM, Paemeleire K, Sacco S, Reuter U, Lampl C, Schytz HW, Katsarava Z, Steiner TJ, Ashina M. Diagnosis and management of migraine in ten steps. Nat Rev Neurol. 2021;17(8):501–14. https://doi.org/10.1038/s41582-021-00509-5.
3. Lipton RB, Stewart WF, Diamond S, Diamond ML, Reed M. Prevalence and burden of migraine in the United States: data from the American Migraine Study II. Headache. 2001;41(7):646–57.
4. Lipton RB, Bigal ME, Diamond M, Freitag F, Reed ML, Stewart WF, AMPP Advisory Group. Migraine prevalence, disease burden, and the need for preventive therapy. Neurology. 2007;68(5):343–9.
5. Vetvik KG, MacGregor EA. Sex differences in the epidemiology, clinical features, and pathophysiology of migraine. Lancet Neurol. 2017;16(1):76–87. https://doi.org/10.1016/S1474-4422(16)30293-9.
6. GBD 2015 DALYs and HALE Collaborators. Global, regional, and national disability-adjusted life-years (DALYs) for 315 diseases and injuries and healthy life expectancy (HALE), 1990–2015: a systematic analysis for the Global Burden of Disease Study 2015. Lancet. 2016;388:1603–58. https://doi.org/10.1016/S0140-6736(16)31460-X.
7. Buse DC, Rupnow MF, Lipton RB. Assessing and managing all aspects of migraine: migraine attacks, migraine-related functional impairment, common comorbidities, and quality of life. Mayo Clin Proc. 2009;84(5):422–35. https://doi.org/10.1016/S0025-6196(11)60561-2.

8. Latinovic R, Gulliford M, Ridsdale L. Headache and migraine in primary care: consultation, prescription, and referral rates in a large population. J Neurol Neurosurg Psychiatry. 2006;77(3):385–7.

9. Alpuente A, Tassorelli C, Diener HC, Silberstein SD, Pozo-Rosich P. Have the IHS guidelines for controlled trials of acute treatment of migraine attacks been followed? Laying the ground for the 4th edition. Cephalalgia. 2020;40(8):778–87. https://doi.org/10.1177/0333102420906843.

10. Headache Classification Committee of the International Headache Society (IHS). The International Classification of Headache Disorders, 3rd edition. Cephalalgia. 2018;38(1):1–211. https://doi.org/10.1177/0333102417738202.

11. https://www.sisc.it/upload/Linee-Guida-Cefalee-Parte-1-1421315319650-4221.pdf

12. Mitsikostas DD, Ashina M, Craven A, Diener HC, Goadsby PJ, Ferrari MD, Lampl C, Paemeleire K, Pascual J, Siva A, Olesen J, Osipova V, Martelletti P. European Headache Federation consensus on technical investigation for primary headache disorders. J Headache Pain. 2015;17:5. https://doi.org/10.1186/s10194-016-0596-y.

13. Metso TM, Tatlisumak T, Debette S, Dallongeville J, Engelter ST, Lyrer PA, Thijs V, Bersano A, Abboud S, Leys D, Grond Ginsbach C, Kloss M, Touzé E, Pezzini A, Metso AJ, CADISP Group. Migraine in cervical artery dissection and ischemic stroke patients. Neurology. 2012;78:1221–8.

14. Joubert J. Diagnosing headache. Aust Fam Physician. 2005;34(8):621–5.

15. Becker WJ, Findlay T, Moga C, Scott NA, Harstall C, Taenzer P. Guideline for primary care management of headache in adults. Can Fam Physician. 2015;61(8):670–9.

16. Simmaco M, Borro M, Missori S, Martelletti P. Pharmacogenomics in migraine: catching biomarkers for predictable disease control. Expert Rev Neurother. 2009;9(9):1267–9.

17. Belyaeva II, Subbotina AG, Eremenko II, Tarasov VV, Chubarev VN, Schiöth HB, Mwinyi J. Pharmacogenetics in primary headache disorders. Front Pharmacol. 2021;12:820214. eCollection 2021. https://doi.org/10.3389/fphar.2021.820214.

18. Steiner TJ, Jensen R, Katsarava Z, Linde M, MacGregor EA, Osipova V, Paemeleire K, Olesen J, Peters M, Martelletti P. Aids to management of headache disorders in primary care (2nd edition): on behalf of the European Headache Federation and Lifting the Burden: the Global Campaign against Headache. J Headache Pain. 2019;20(1):57. https://doi.org/10.1186/s10194-018-0899-2.

19. Tassorelli C, Diener HC, Dodick DW, et al. Guidelines of the International Headache Society for controlled trials of preventive treatment of chronic migraine in adults. Cephalalgia. 2018;38:815–32.

20. Diener HC, Tassorelli C, Dodick DW, et al. Guidelines of the International Headache Society for controlled trials of acute treatment of migraine attacks in adults: fourth edition. Cephalalgia. 2019;39:687–710.

21. Do TP, Guo S, Ashina M. Therapeutic novelties in migraine: new drugs, new hope? J Headache Pain. 2019;20(1):37. https://doi.org/10.1186/s10194-019-0974-3. Erratum in: J Headache Pain. 2019 May 17;20(1):55

22. Moreno-Ajona D, Pérez-Rodríguez A, Goadsby PJ. Gepants, calcitonin-gene-related peptide receptor antagonists: what could be their role in migraine treatment? Curr Opin Neurol. 2020;33(3):309–15. https://doi.org/10.1097/WCO.0000000000000806.

23. Lipton RB, Dodick DW, Ailani J, Lu K, Finnegan M, Szegedi A, Trugman JM. Effect of ubrogepant vs placebo on pain and the most bothersome associated symptom in the acute treatment of migraine: the ACHIEVE II randomized clinical trial. JAMA. 2019;322(19):1887–98. https://doi.org/10.1001/jama.2019.16711. Erratum in: JAMA. 2020 Apr 7;323(13):1318

24. Martelletti P, Luciani M, Spuntarelli V, Bentivegna E. Deprescribing in migraine. Expert Opin Drug Saf. 2021;20(6):623–5. https://doi.org/10.1080/14740338.2021.1907342.

25. IHS. Guidelines for controlled trials of drugs in migraine. First edition. International Headache Society Committee on Clinical Trials in Migraine. Cephalalgia. 1991;11:1–12.

26. Mitsikostas DD, Belesioti I, Arvaniti C, et al. Patients' preferences for headache acute and preventive treatment. J Headache Pain. 2017;18:102.

27. Tfelt-Hansen P, Pascual J, Ramadan N, Dahlöf C, Damico D, Diener H-C, et al. Guidelines for controlled trials of drugs in migraine: third edition. A guide for investigators. Cephalalgia. 2012;32(1):6–38.
28. Macedo A, Farré M, Baños JE. A meta-analysis of the placebo response in acute migraine and how this response may be influenced by some of the characteristics of clinical trials. Eur J Clin Pharmacol. 2006;62(3):161–72. https://doi.org/10.1007/s00228-005-0088-5.
29. International Council for Harmonisation of Technical Requirements for Pharmaceuticals for Human Use. Guideline for good clinical practice. https://www.ich.org/fileadmin/Public_Web_Site/ICH_Products/Guidelines/Efficacy/E6/E6_R1_Guideline.pdf. Accessed 29 May 2017.
30. International Committee of Medical Journal Editors. Defining the role of authors and contributors. http://www.icmje.org/recommendations/browse/roles-and-responsibilities/defining-the-role-of-authors-and-contributors.html. Accessed 25 Nov 2018.
31. Diener H-C, Tassorelli C, Diener H-C, Dodick DW, International Headache Society Clinical Trials Committee, et al. Guidelines of the International Headache Society for controlled trials of preventive treatment of migraine attacks in episodic migraine adults. Cephalalgia. 2020;40(10):1026–44.
32. Diener H-C, Tassorelli C, Diener H-C, Dodick DW, International Headache Society Clinical Trials Standing Committee, et al. Guidelines of the International Headache Society for controlled trials of preventive treatment of migraine attacks in episodic migraine adults. Cephalalgia. 2018;38(5):815–32.

# Chapter 2
# Clinical Scales for Headache and Migraine

Pınar Yalınay Dikmen and Betul Baykan

## 2.1 Introduction

Headache is a very common condition for mankind. About half of the adult population have had a headache at least once within the past year [1]. Indeed, headache disorders are very frequent and characterized by recurrent headache attacks as well as associated symptoms. These disorders are related to personal and societal burdens of pain, disability, reduced quality of life, increased usage of medical services and financial cost. Despite their high prevalences, headache disorders are still underdiagnosed and undertreated. Only a minority of patients with headache disorders are diagnosed by a healthcare provider. In fact, many patients with headaches have been managed by non-headache specialist health care professionals, generally in primary care [2].

Patient-related outcome measures (PROMs) are defined by the U.S. Food and Drug Administration (FDA) as any reports of the status of a patient's health condition that comes directly from the patient, without interpretation of the patient's response by a clinician or anyone else [3]. PROMs also endorse the reporting of health measurement instruments (COSMIN statement), the diagnostic accuracy studies (STARD statement), systematic reviews (PRISMA statement), observational studies in epidemiology (STROBE statement), studies conducted using observational routinely collected health data (RECORD statement) [4–9]. PROMs aim to provide a patient-based assessment of the impact of headache on how people feel, function, and live their lives. Many PROMs are used in headache trials to

P. Yalınay Dikmen (✉)
Department of Neurology, School of Medicine, Acıbadem University, Istanbul, Turkey
e-mail: pinar.yalinay@acibadem.edu.tr

B. Baykan
Department of Neurology, Istanbul Faculty of Medicine, Istanbul University, Istanbul, Turkey
e-mail: baykanb@istanbul.edu.tr



P. Yalınay Dikmen, A. Özge (eds.), *Clinical Scales for Headache Disorders*, Headache, https://doi.org/10.1007/978-3-031-25938-8_2

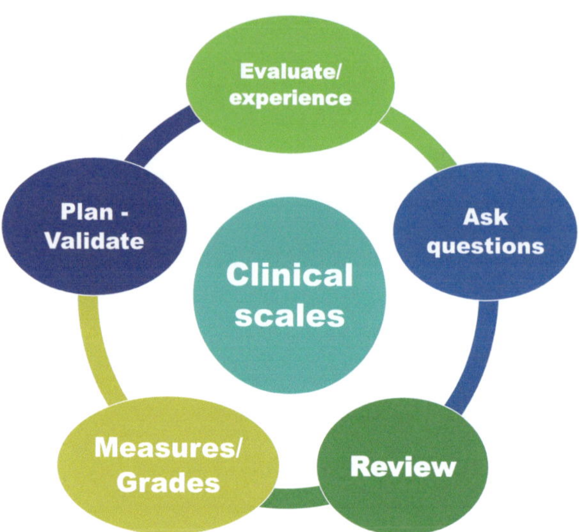

**Fig. 2.1** Headache disorders can be measured with clinical scales



assess headache or migraine impact, health or migraine-related quality of life, associated symptoms (like allodynia, nausea), psychiatric comorbidities and cognitive processes, treatment monitoring and optimization.

The main aim of these clinical scales is not different from other kinds of measurement tools in research and clinical settings. They ask questions, measure grades or levels, evaluate the available evidence, and plan further improvements after gaining experiences (Fig. 2.1). In this chapter, PROMs and clinical scales used in headache disorders as well as in migraine will be briefly introduced to readers. Then, they will be explained and discussed in detail throughout the following chapters of this book.

## 2.2 Diagnostic Screeners for Headache and Migraine (Table 2.1)

### 2.2.1 SNOOP

Recently published Consensus Statement provided a ten-steps approach to the diagnosis and management of migraine [10]. For a diagnosis of migraine, the Consensus Statement suggests recording medical history, applying diagnostic criteria, considering differential diagnosis, examining the patient to exclude other causes, and using neuroimaging only when a secondary headache disorder is suspected. General practitioners (GP) mostly play a major role in the diagnosis, management, and treatment of headache. GPs are usually the first physician to evaluate a patient with a headache. After that, GPs decide to manage the patient or refer the patient to a neurologist. Neurologists use International Classification Headache Disorders-3

**Table 2.1**  Diagnostic screeners for headache disorders and migraine help clinicians

| |
|---|
| **SNOOP** is a diagnostic screen developed for secondary headaches. |
| **ID Migraine™** was created as a screening instrument for migraine. |
| **The Erwin Test** is a three-item brief diagnostic instrument for cluster headaches. |
| **The Brief Headache Screen (BHS)** is a four-item, self-administered screening tool for migraine and chronic daily headache and medication overuse headache. |
| **Migraine Screen Questionnaire (MS-Q)** is a self-administered questionnaire for the screening of migraine. |
| **The Computerized Headache Assessment Tool (CHAT)** was created for the diagnosis of primary headache, making the distinction between episodic and chronic daily headache, and capturing medication overuse headache. |
| **The Headache Under-Response to Treatment (HURT)** is an eight-item, self-administered questionnaire with five domains as follows: headache frequency, headache-related disability, acute medication use, perceived control of headaches and knowledge and the understanding of diagnosis. |

**Table 2.2**  Red flags might be remembered by the mnemonic, SNOOP [12]

| |
|---|
| **S**ystemic symptoms or illness (including fever, persistent or progressive vomiting, stiff neck, pregnancy, cancer, immunocompromised state, and anticoagulation), |
| **N**eurological signs and symptoms (including altered mental status, focal neurological symptoms or signs, seizures or papilledema), |
| **O**nset is new (especially in those age 40 years or older) or sudden, |
| **O**ther associated conditions (e.g., headache is after head trauma, awakens patient from sleep, or is worsened by Valsalva maneuvers), |
| **P**rior headache history that is different (e.g., headaches now are of a different pattern or are rapidly progressive in severity or frequency. |

(ICHD) criteria for headache diagnosis to exclude secondary headache and to diagnose the specific primary headache disorder [11]. However, GP might not be familiar with ICHD-3 criteria. For that reason many screening instruments have been developed to diagnose headache disorders as well as the exclusion of secondary reasons of headache. In the primary care population, excluding secondary headache has a critical importance. SNOOP is widely used as a diagnostic screener for secondary headache (Table 2.2) [12].

### 2.2.2  ID Migraine™

ID Migraine™ (IDM™) has been known as a well-validated, reliable, and efficient screening tool for migraine (Table 2.3) [13]. In the primary care setting, a subset of three questions (disabling headache, nausea, and sensitivity to light) ensured optimum performance. IDM™ showed, with two out of three questions as a positive result, a sensitivity of 0.81 and a specificity of 0.75, and a positive predictive value of 0.93. It has been translated and validated for use in several languages. Moreover, IDM™ is extensively used and validated in many settings including workplaces and ophthalmology and ENT clinics [14–16].

**Table 2.3** IDM™ can efficiently help to show that a patient's headache is likely a migraine with the following three questions

1. Has a headache limited your activities for a day or more in the last 3 months?
2. Are you nauseated or sick to your stomach when you have a headache?
3. Does light bother you when you have a headache?

**Table 2.4** The Erwin Test for cluster headache is a promising screening tool

1. Is this the worst pain you ever experienced? Yes, No
2. Imagine a setting timer. Does the headache last less than 4 h? Yes, No
3. During a headache, do one or more of these happen to you? Yes, No
…Your eye turns red on only one side
…Your eye waters on only one side,
…Your nose runs on only one side
…Your nose gets congested on only one side

### 2.2.3 The Erwin Test for Cluster Headache

The Erwin Test for Cluster Headache is a three-item brief diagnostic tool [17] (Table 2.4). A study showed that three items had a high sensitivity of 84% (95% confidence interval (CI): 73–92%), a high specificity of 89 (95% CI: 84–94%) as well as positive predictive value of 76% (95% CI 64–85%), and negative predictive value of 93% (95% CI: 88–97%) for the diagnosis of cluster headache (CH) in 224 patients. Three items of The Ervin Test explore headache intensity, duration and associated autonomic features. However, it has not been validated in a large clinical headache population to date.

### 2.2.4 The Brief Headache Screen (BHS)

The BHS is a four-item, self-administered instrument that screens effectively not only for migraine but also for chronic daily headache (CDH) and medication overuse headache (MOH) [18]. The BHS has shown 82.6% agreement with IDM™ (95% CI: 77.8–87.4%) [19].

In question 1, the frequency of severe (disabling) headache is asked to screen for migraine if the frequency of severe (disabling) headache is at least once per month to once per year.

In question 2, the severity of headache (mild or less severe) is evaluated to detect CDH.

In question 3, MOH is captured.

Finally, question 4 aims to evaluate headache-related disability.

### 2.2.5  Migraine Screen Questionnaire (MS-Q)

The MS-Q is a five-item instrument with a sensitivity of 0.93, a specificity of 0.81 and a positive predictive value of 0.83 [20]. The MS-Q was also validated in the primary care setting to detect hidden migraine [21].

### 2.2.6  The Computerized Headache Assessment Tool (CHAT)

The CHAT is an expert system for diagnosing primary headache disorders, making the distinction between episodic, chronic, and daily ones and capturing MOH [22].

### 2.2.7  The Headache Under-Response to Treatment (HURT)

The HURT questionnaire was created by an expert consensus group as a part of the non-government organization "Lifting the Burden" (LTB) [23]. The HURT is intended to combine both an assessment of headache and decision-making for better headache management. Authors declared that no single instrument covers many aspects of the care for primary headache disorders until the HURT and there is a need for a simple but comprehensive instrument to guide and monitor the treatment of primary headache disorders. It has an eight-item, self-administered questionnaire addressing five domains as follows: headache frequency, headache-related disability, acute medication use, perceived control of headaches and knowledge and the understanding of diagnosis.

## 2.3  Scales for Impact, Disability, and Burden of Headache and Migraine (Table 2.5)

### 2.3.1  Headache Specific Impact

#### 2.3.1.1  Headache Impact Test (HIT-6)

The HIT-6 is a widely used PROM to evaluate the impact of headache on an individual's functional health and well-being [24]. This six-item questionnaire with powerful psychometric validation against a large item pool can discriminate robustly between migraine and non-migraine headache. It is easy to use and score. It is made up of six items to assess the frequency of severe headache, limitations of daily activities (including work, school, and leisure time), desire to lie down, fatigue, irritability, and difficulty concentrating. A total sum score is between 36 and 78. The

**Table 2.5** Clinical scales and PROMs related to impact, disability, and burden of headache

| |
|---|
| **Headache Impact Test (HIT-6)** is a six-item questionnaire that aims to assess the impact of headache on functional health and well-being of patients. |
| **Headache-Attributed Lost Time (HALT-90) Index** is used for migraine as well as an evaluation of headache-related lost productive time for all headache disorders within the past 3 months. |
| **Headache-Attributed Lost Time (HALT-30) Index** was created keeping the same structure as HALT-90 for an assessment of the previous 30 days. |
| **Headache-Attributed Lost Time (HALT-7) Index** was created keeping the same structure as HALT-90 for an assessment of the previous 7 days. |
| **Henry Ford Headache Disability Inventory (HDI)** is a 25-item questionnaire for measuring both ictal and interictal burden of headache. The Spouse HDI is like the HDI, "I" was changed to "my spouse". |
| **Headache Impact Questionnaire (HImQ)** is a 16-item questionnaire regarding (paid work, housework, and non-work activities) headache duration, pain intensity, need for bed rest, and disability in three domains within the previous 3 months. |
| **Cluster Headache Impact Questionnaire (CHIQ)** is an eight-item questionnaire used to evaluate cluster headache-related disability in the last week. |
| **Headache-Attributed Restriction, Disability, Social Handicap, and Impaired Participation (HARDSHIP) Questionnaire** was developed to assess the burden of primary headaches for the EUROLIGHT project [39]. HARDSHIP has a well-developed multi-modular design as follows: demographic module, screen module, frequent headache module (>15 days/month), diagnostic module, sensitivities and specificities of the HARDSHIP diagnostic questions, for migraine as well as tension-type headache, health-resource utilization module, disability module, module on headache of yesterday, module on interictal burden, module on quality of life, module on subjective well-being, module on perception control, module on overall burden (willing-to-pay), module on cumulative burden (impact on education, career and earnings) and lastly HARDSHIP module on burden on others, including partner and children. |
| **Headache Activities of Daily Living Index (HADLI)** is a nine-item questionnaire exclusively composed of items on specific headache-related activities of daily living as follows: ability to work, socialize, travel, read, drive, personal care, lift, sleep, exercise, and recreation. |
| **Headache Disability Questionnaire (HDQ)** is a nine-item questionnaire used as a headache-specific disability survey intended for use in patients under physiotherapy for their headaches. |
| **Headache Needs Assessment Survey (HANA)** is a seven-item survey that was designed to evaluate the frequency and the most bothersome symptom due to migraine, as well as other types of headaches. |

impact scores are classified as little or no impact (grade 1: score 36–49), moderate impact (grade 2: score 50–55), substantial impact (grade 3: score 56–59) or severe impact (grade 4: score 60–78) [25]. The HIT-6 is translated into several languages including Turkish and showed strong evidence of reliability and validity [26].

From a practical point of view, the HIT-6 score is taken at baseline and then every 4 weeks after treatment and could be used as a reliable indicator of the response to the treatment [25]. PROM score interpretation needs guidance on what change in score means a meaningful change in "headache" for the individual patient (minimal important change (MIC)) and what difference means a meaningful difference between groups of patients defined by some external marker (minimal important difference (MID)) [27, 28]. Regarding MID for the HIT-6, a decline of 2.3 points in total score after treatment shows a clinically substantial improvement in patients with chronic daily headache [29]. The between-group MID (defined as the smallest difference in scores between groups that patients comprehend as important or helpful) for the HIT-6 is a 1.5-point reduction (−1.5) [30].

### 2.3.1.2 Headache-Attributed Lost Time (HALT-90) Index

The HALT-90 is also created by the LTB and is a direct derivative of MIDAS, but not specifically for migraine but also it can be used for an evaluation of headache-related lost productive time to all headache disorders within the preceding 3 months [31]. It has been validated in epidemiological studies rather than in clinical settings. It measures only ictal disability. A total score of HALT-90 is classified as grade I, minimal or no infrequent impact (score of 0–5); grade II, mild or infrequent impact (score of 6–10); grade III (indicates high need for care), moderate impact (score of 11–20); and grade IV (indicates high need for care), severe impact (score of ≥21)

Then, two alternative forms of HALT were created keeping the same structure (**HALT-7/30**) for an assessment of different periods [32]. HALT-7/30 serves, both for an assessment of lost and productive time (work time, household work time, social events) with overcoming recall bias. HALT-30 might be more easily applicable in follow-up treatment measurements. In the special setting of a work-based clinic in Turkey, employees who reported headaches on ≥10 days/month were just 2.9% of the workforce but accounted for 36.9% of headache-related productivity losses [33]. In that way, HALT enables an evaluation of disability as well as a lost productive time and a secondary burden of financial cost.

### 2.3.1.3 Henry Ford Headache Disability Inventory (HDI)

The HDI is developed to measure the burden of recurrent headaches on activities of daily living [34, 35]. It is a 25-item questionnaire for measuring both ictal and interictal burdens of headache. It has two subdomains regarding functional and emotional impairment. The highest score of 100 indicates the highest disability level. The HDI has strong test-retest reliability at 2 months (Pearson's r = 0.83) as well as at 1 week (Pearson's r = 0.93). The Spouse HDI is identical to the HDI, "I" substitutes with "my spouse". It also has high convent validity with the respondent spouse's observations of the headache-related quality of life (QoL) (Pearson's r = 0.78). Indeed, the HDI is a useful research tool, but it is hard to integrate into the clinical setting because of partly difficult to score as well as it is not obvious how it informs treatment [23, 36].

### 2.3.1.4 Headache Impact Questionnaire (HImQ)

The HImQ is a 16-item questionnaire, related to headache duration, pain intensity, need for bed rest and disability in three domains (paid work, housework and non-work activities [37]. The HImQ resembles MIDAS but it combines measures of both pain and disability into a single-scaled measure of severity to evaluate the collective impact of headache on an individual in the previous 3 months. Scoring is somewhat complex; many steps involving multiplication and addition are needed to get a total summed score. However, it is more precise than MIDAS for measuring the impact of other headache disorders (e.g. CH). It has a good test-retest validity (average Pearson's r = 0.77). Moreover, the HImQ showed a moderate convergent validity with a 90-day daily diary (Pearson's r = 0.49).

### 2.3.1.5 Cluster Headache Impact Questionnaire (CHIQ)

The CHIQ is developed as a short measure of CH-related disability. The CHIQ was created based on a literature review and interviews with patients and experts by a German support group [38]. The CHIQ is an eight-item questionnaire with a good consistency (Cronbach's α = 0.88) and a test-retest reliability (ICC 0.91, n = 41). In validation, the CHIQ showed significant correlations with the HIT-6 (r = 0.58, p < 0.001), subscales of the depression, anxiety and stress scales (DASS) (r = 0.46–0.62; p < 0.001) as well as with CH' attack frequency (r = 0.41; p < 0.001). Furthermore, this short CH-specific disability questionnaire was able to differentiate between chronic CH (n = 111), active episodic CH (n = 85) and episodic CH patients (n = 52) in remission (p < 0.05 for all three comparisons).

### 2.3.1.6 Headache-Attributed Restriction, Disability, Social Handicap and Impaired Participation (HARDSHIP) Questionnaire

The HARDSHIP questionnaire is created to evaluate the burden of primary headache disorders in Europe for EUROLIGHT project [39]. This questionnaire has a multi-modular design as follows: demographic module, screen module, frequent headache module (15 or more days/month), diagnostic module, sensitivities and specificities of the HARDSHIP diagnostic questions set, for migraine and tension-type headache, health-resource utilization module, disability module, HARDSHIP module on headache of yesterday, HARDSHIP module on interictal burden, HARDSHIP module on quality of life, HARDSHIP module on subjective well-being, HARDSHIP module on perception control, HARDSHIP module on overall burden (willing-to-pay), HARDSHIP module on cumulative burden (impact on education, career and earnings) and HARDSHIP module on burden on others (household partner and children).

The modules within the HARDSHIP questionnaire cover symptom burden, treatment, and health-resource utilization, disability and productive time losses, interictal burden, quality of life and subjective well-being, perception control, overall individual burden (willingness to pay for treatment as a summary measure), cumulative burden (impact on education, career and earnings), effects on relationships, love life and family dynamics, burden on others, including household partner and children and financial cost [40]. The HARDSHIP questionnaire has undergone testing in 20 countries and 19 languages, and it is constrained by ICHD-3 [11]. However, the reliability and validity of HARDSHIP questionnaire is unknown and therefore, thought as limited.

### 2.3.1.7  Headache Activities of Daily Living Index (HADLI)

The HADLI is created to assess specific activities of daily living (ADL) [41]. Indeed, various widely used instruments have items not only associated with specific ADL but also severity of pain, quality of life, symptoms, etc. The HADLI is a nine-item questionnaire exclusively composed of items on specific headache-related ADL as follows: ability to work, socialize, traveling, reading, driving, personal care, lifting, sleep, exercising and recreation. On the other hand, the HADLI has a limited internal consistency and a limited content validity [42].

### 2.3.1.8  Headache Disability Questionnaire (HDQ)

The HDQ is a nine-item questionnaire for use in physiotherapy clinics [43]. The aim of creation of HDQ is to develop items for a headache-specific disability questionnaire suitable for patients receiving physiotherapy treatment for their headaches, but not specifically migraine. Nine items of the HDQ cover three domains as follows: pain severity, prevention of activity and reduction in ability to perform activity. The HDQ has a limited internal consistency and a limited structural validity [42].

### 2.3.1.9  Headache Needs Assessment Survey (HANA)

The HANA is a seven-item questionnaire that is designed to evaluate "frequency" and "bothersome symptoms" because of migraine and it is also applicable to other types of headaches [44]. The items are regarding anxiety/worry, depression/discouragement, self-control, energy, function/work, family/social activities, and overall impact on a patient's life. The HANA showed a good test-retest reliability (Pearson's r = 0.78) and a good correlation with HDI scores (r = 0.73, p < 0.0001).

**Table 2.6** Clinical scales and PROMs related to impact, disability, and burden of migraine

| |
|---|
| **Migraine Severity (MIGSEV) Scale** is a seven-item self-assessment questionnaire used to evaluate migraine severity. |
| **Migraine Disability Assessment Questionnaire (MIDAS)** evaluates absenteeism and presentism in work/school, household work and family/social activities because of migraine in the past 3 months. |
| **The Pediatric Migraine Disability Assessment Score (PedMIDAS)** was created keeping the same structure as MIDAS for evaluating headache disability and the impact of migraine headaches in children and adolescents. |
| **Functional Assessment in Migraine (FAIM) Questionnaire** measures the impact of migraine on mental functioning and activity and participation. |
| **Migraine Interictal Burden Scale-4 (MIBS-4)** is a four-item, self-administrated survey for the measurement of interictal migraine-related burden of the four following areas: impairments in the workplace or school, impairments in the social life, family, problems making plans or commitments, and emotional/affective and cognitive stress. |
| **Migraine Functional Impact Questionnaire (MFIQ)** is a 26-item self-report questionnaire that was created to address the compressive impact of migraine in the past 7 days on Physical Function (PF), Usual Activities (UA), Social Function (SF) and Emotional Function (EF). |

## *2.3.2 Migraine Specific Impact (Table 2.6)*

### 2.3.2.1 Migraine Severity (MIGSEV) Scale

The MIGSEV is a seven-item questionnaire to design for a measurement of migraine severity [45]. The MIGSEV has three domains:

1. Intensity of attacks,
2. Frequency of attacks,
3. Resistance to treatment.

The MIGSEV has been demonstrated as a suitable questionnaire to measure for migraine severity in a large prospective survey [46]. It has a capacity to show a relationship between migraine severity and quality of life in patients with migraine. Therefore the MIGSEV is recommended to both physicians and patients for an assessment of migraine severity.

### 2.3.2.2 Migraine Disability Assessment Questionnaire (MIDAS)

The MIDAS is a five-item questionnaire and was developed by Steward WF et al. in 1999 [47, 48]. Since then MIDAS is a widely used tool to detect as well as to follow-up disability in patients with migraine. The MIDAS evaluates absenteeism and presentism in days of work/school, household work and family/social activities within the past 3 months. A total score is graded as grade I, little or no disability (score of 0–5); grade II, mild disability (score of 6–10); grade III, moderate disability (score of 11–20); and grade IV, severe disability (score of ≥21) (S43). The MIDAS is one of the commonly used PROMs with the HIT-6 in headache clinical studies [42]. The MIDAS has been validated across many countries and translated into many different languages. Indeed, it measures just the ictal burden of migraine, but not the interictal burden. Two additional questions (MIDAS A and B) evaluate pain frequency and pain intensity within the last 3 months, respectively. The between-group minimally important difference for MIDAS is a five-point reduction (−5) [49].

### 2.3.2.3  Functional Assessment in Migraine (FAIM) Questionnaire

The FAIM was created by the World Health Organization International Classification of Impairments, Disabilities, and Handicaps, version 2 (ICHD-2) [50]. The FAIM has a moderate internal consistency (Cronbach's $\alpha > 0.70$) and a moderate structural validity (positive correlation with the Migraine Specific QoL (MSQoL) questionnaire (0.20–0.51)).

This questionnaire has three main domains:

1. Body structure and function, including mental functioning,
2. Activity,
3. Participation.

### 2.3.2.4  Migraine Interictal Burden Scale-4 (MIBS-4)

The MIBS-4 is a four-item, self-administrated questionnaire with five Likert-type response options plus "don't know/not available-NA" for a measurement of burden associated with migraine between the attacks [51]. The MIBS-4 measures interictal migraine-related burden in four dimensions:

1. Impairment in work or school,
2. Impairment in family and social life,
3. Difficulty in making plans or commitments,
4. Emotional/affective and cognitive stress.

Responses to each question are multiplied to get a total sum score showing one of four levels of interictal burden of migraine: none, mild, moderate, or severe. When interictal burden increases, quality of life reduces, understandably. It is validated against MIDAS (Spearman $r = 0.40$), HIT-6 (Spearman $r = 0.44$), PHQ-9 (Spearman $r = 0.41$) and MSQoL (Spearman $r = 0.40$) [52]. A moderate negative correlation was found between MIBS-4 and MSQ (total score ($r = 0.48$) and its subscales. Indeed, ictal burden only partially predicts an impact of burden because of migraine. In addition to that it increases rates of psychiatric comorbidities in patients with migraine [53].

### 2.3.2.5  Migraine Functional Impact Questionnaire (MFIQ)

The MFIQ is a novel PROM and a 26-item self-report questionnaire. The MFIQ was created following the methods recommended by FDA and by the ISPOR Good Research Practices [54–56]. A range of total score is between 0 and 100. Higher scores on a 0–100 scale indicates greater impact.

The MFIQ was created to address the compressive impact of migraine in the past 7 days on Physical Function (PF), Usual Activities (UA), Social Function (SF) and Emotional Function (EF). This new instrument offers a more comprehensive measurement of the impacts of migraine compared to existing instruments (such as the HIT-6 or MIDAS). The MFIQ has two versions (1 and 2). The MFIQ has been translated into 20 languages following best practice recommendations for linguistic validation of PROM instruments [57]. Furthermore, the MFIQ has been included in the "Guidelines of the International Headache Society for controlled trials of preventive treatment of chronic migraine in adults" as a PROM tool [58].

## 2.4  Scales for Generic and Migraine Specific Health-Related Quality of Life (HRQoL) (Table 2.7)

### 2.4.1  Generic HRQoL Scales

#### 2.4.1.1  Short Form (SF) 36 (SF-36) (SF-12) (SF-8)

The SF-36 comprises 36 questions, as the name indicated and evaluates a range of symptoms related to common diseases [59]. The SF has two more versions, consisting of 12 items and 8 items [60, 61]. It has eight different subscores as

**Table 2.7** Clinical scales and PROMs regarding generic and migraine specific health-related quality of life (HRQoL)

| |
|---|
| **Generic HRQoL Scales** |
| **Short Form 36 (SF-36)** is a 36-item questionnaire that has eight different subscores as follows: physical and social functioning, physical and social role limitations, mental health, energy, pain, and mental summary. |
| **Short Form 12** was created keeping the same structure as the SF-36 for evaluating HRQoL. |
| **Short Form 8** was created keeping the same structure as the SF-36 for evaluating HRQoL. |
| **EuroQoL Quality of Life Scale (EQ-5D)** is a self-reported instrument for the assessment of HRQoL. It has two dimensions as follows: a descriptive system and a visual analog scale. |
| **Migraine Specific HRQoL Scales** |
| **Migraine Specific Quality of Life (MSQ v2.1) version 2.1** is a 14-item questionnaire that evaluates the limitations caused by migraine attacks on social and work-based activities. Three essential dimensions of HRQoL are measured by the MSQ v2.1 as follows: role-function-restrictive, role-function-preventive, and emotional functions with 4-week recall period. |

follows: physical and social functioning, physical and social role limitations, mental health, energy, pain, and mental summary. The maximum score of 100 indicates the best possible health state. Patients with migraine have significantly lower SF-36 scores than individuals without migraine, and migraine adversely affects functioning at least as much as depression, diabetes mellitus, and recent myocardial infarction [62]. Moreover, patients with migraine have lower HRQoL than those in the general population with no chronic diseases [63, 64]. SF-36 has also a modified version for a headache population [65]. In a population based and case-control study, individuals with migraine scored significantly lower than individuals without migraine in eight of the nine HRQoL domains of the SF-36 [66]. The SF-36 and SF-8 have both acceptable evidence of construct validity, whereas evidence for SF-12 is limited in headache population, so far [42].

### 2.4.1.2  EuroQoL Quality of Life Scale (EQ-5D)

The ED-5D is one of the most widely used self-reported instruments for measuring health-related quality of life [67]. It consists of two parts:

1. Part 1 is a descriptive system,
2. Part 2 is a visual analogue scale (VAS)

The Part 1 comprises five single-item dimensions on mobility, self-care, pain/discomfort, usual activities, and psychological status (anxiety/depression) with three possible answers for each item (1 = no problem), (2 = moderate problem), and (3 = severe problem). On the other hand, Part 2 uses a vertical graduated VAS (thermometer) to measure health status, ranging from worst imaginable health state to best imaginable health state. The score of 1 indicates the best health state, whereas higher scores indicate more severe and frequent problems. Studies about health utilities are beneficial for understanding the general chronic burden of migraine in the population. Evidence for reliability, validity, and construct validity of the EQ-5D in headache population was limited [42, 68].

## 2.4.2  Migraine Specific HRQoL Scales

### 2.4.2.1  Migraine Specific Quality of Life (MSQ v2.1) Version 2.1

The MSQ v2.1 is a 14-item PROM instrument that has three domains about the limitations caused by migraine attacks on daily social and work-related activities [69, 70]. These three essential dimensions of HRQoL are measured by MSQ as follows: role-function-restrictive (RR, seven items), role-function-preventive (RP, four items) and emotional functions (EF, three items) with 4-week recall period. Each item is responded by using six-point scale: "none of the time", "a little bit of the time", "some of the time", "a good bit of the time", "most of the time" and "all the time", which are assigned scores of 1–6, respectively. Higher scores of MSQ indicates better migraine-related quality of life. Regarding the cut points of between-group minimal differences for MSQ domains, MSQ-RFR, MSQ-RFP, MSQ-EF are (3.2-), (4.6-) and (7.5-) points, respectively [71].

The MSQ is a widely used PROM to quantify the potential benefits of treatment in clinical studies of migraine [72]. The conceptual framework of the MSQ was created from an expert review of the migraine literature and it was validated in a sample of 458 patients with migraine. The psychometric properties of the MSQ were also studied in patients with chronic migraine and was shown as a valid tool to reliably measure the impact of migraine among those patients [73].

## 2.5 Scales for Treatment Monitoring and Optimization of Headache and Migraine (Table 2.8)

### 2.5.1 Completeness of Response to Migraine Therapy (CORS)

The CORS is one of the six PROMs evaluating response to or satisfaction with migraine specific treatments [74]. Both from the perspective of headache experts and patients, CORS evaluates burden of migraine, cognition, and difficulty with thinking as well as confidence in/or satisfaction with treatment options.

**Table 2.8** Instruments and PROMs with treatment monitoring and optimization for headache and migraine

| |
|---|
| **Completeness of Response to migraine therapy (CORS)** has two main modules. The static CORS delicately evaluates satisfaction with migraine specific one treatment. The second comparative CORS indicates a more general comparison between two treatments. All modules aim to reveal unmet needs and improvements during research or a clinical setting in patients under migraine treatment. |
| **Migraine Assessment of Current Therapy (Migraine-ACT)** has four dichotomic (yes or no) questions to evaluate satisfaction with treatment, whether acute treatment is successful or needs modification. |
| **Migraine-Treatment Assessment Questionnaire (M-TAQ)** is a nine-item self-reported questionnaire used to detect management problems and determine individuals with suboptimal migraine management in the primary care setting. |
| **Migraine-Treatment Optimization Questionnaire (M-TOQ)** was created as a long form for use in research settings (M-TOQ-15) and a short form for use in primary care (M-TOQ-5). M-TOQ aims to evaluate five domains as follows: functioning, rapid relief, consistency of relief, risk of recurrence and tolerability with migraine treatment. |
| **Migraine-Treatment Satisfaction Measure (MTSM)** was created in 2003, aiming to disclose the gap between the patients' expectations before and after a given treatment. |
| **Patient Perception of Migraine Questionnaire-Revised (PPMQ-R)** is a 32-item questionnaire used to measure patient satisfaction in terms of acute migraine management comprising efficacy, functionality, ease of use, cost, and tolerability scales. |

The CORS has two main modules. First, the static CORS, which comprehensively assessed one treatment, whereas the second comparative CORS provides a more global comparison between two treatments at a particular time point. All modules aim to measure unmet needs and improvements during research or in a clinical setting. The CORS has a high but a limited internal consistency (alpha range: 0.88–0.94). In terms of validity, the CORS has moderate content validity, limited structural and construct validities [42]. CORS has the ability to demonstrate the superiority of new migraine therapies over traditional ones. Indeed, the CORS aims to detect the resolution of headache pain and patients' return to normal functioning. The CORS also provides comparison of two migraine therapies simultaneously in different settings.

### 2.5.2  Migraine Assessment of Current Therapy (Migraine-ACT)

The Migraine-ACT has four dichotomic (yes or no) questions to assess satisfaction with treatment whether acute treatment is effective or requires modification (Table 2.9) [75]. Migraine-ACT was created by headache experts and researchers and has acceptable evidence of temporal stability and unknown validity. Migraine-ACT evaluates impact, global assessment of relief, consistency of response and emotional response. A single "no" response means that there is no need for doing any modification in acute treatment. Migraine-ACT is an easy and a useful tool for evaluating the effectiveness of acute therapy.

### 2.5.3  Migraine-Treatment Assessment Questionnaire (M-TAQ)

The M-TAQ is a nine-item self-reported questionnaire to detect management problems and to identify individuals whose migraine management may be suboptimal in a primary care setting [76]. The M-TAQ has a limited temporal stability, content validity and construct validity [42]. It may be used to screen a population of migraineurs for suboptimal management. It should be kept in mind that the MTAQ is not reliable enough to be used alone in making decisions regarding individual migraine management [77]. Depending on the sensitivity and specificity

**Table 2.9** Migraine-ACT evaluates whether acute treatment is effective or requires modification

| When you take treatment: |
| --- |
| 1. Does your migraine medication work consistently, in a majority of attacks? |
| 2. Does your headache pain disappear within 2 h? |
| 3. Are you able to function normally within 2 h? |
| 4. Are you comfortable enough with your medication to be able to plan your daily activities? |

of the modified total MTAQ score to predict suboptimal management, a score of 2 is recommended as a cutoff point for additional follow-up. This allows for a reasonably high level of sensitivity, indicating detection of those migraineurs who are inadequately managed; however, this cut-off value has a low level of specificity, indicating patients who are appropriately managed but whose MTAQ score would indicate the need for follow-up. Additional analyses are needed to confirm the MTAQ's psychometric properties in larger and diverse migraine populations, and to improve the questionnaire's generalizability [78].

### 2.5.4   Migraine-Treatment Optimization Questionnaire (M-TOQ)

The M-TOQ was created as a long-version for the use in research (M-TOQ-15) and as a short-version for use in primary care (M-TOQ-5). The validation and reliability study of MTOQ was conducted in a total of 25 primary care centers and it is validated in five languages (English, French, German, Italian and Spanish). It has a limited internal consistency and a limited temporal stability for reliability [79]. Content and structural validities of the M-TOQ were also limited. The MTOQ aims to evaluate five treatment optimization domains as follows, functioning, rapid relief, consistency of relief, risk of recurrence and tolerability. The Cronbach alpha for M-TOQ-15 was 0.85, and it correlated well with MIDAS, HIT-6 and MSQoL ($r = 0.33$–$0.44$). The Cronbach alpha for M-TOQ-5 was 0.66, and it also correlated well with the three questionnaires ($r = 0.33$–$0.41$). However, the recommendation for a utility of the M-TOQ for evaluating treatment benefit in research (M-TOQ-15) and clinical practice (M-TOQ-5) should be further validated.

### 2.5.5   Migraine-Treatment Satisfaction Measure (MTSM)

The MTSM was created in 2003 by Patrick et al., aiming to disclose a gap between the patients' expectation before and after a given treatment [80]. A purpose of pilot study was to generate a small experimental data set to develop and assess the potential usefulness of the conceptual model and scoring algorithm for this application of a new measurement strategy. The MTSM had a limited reliability and a limited validity. Hence further validation is warranted.

## *2.5.6   Patient Perception of Migraine Questionnaire-Revised (PPMQ-R)*

The PPMQ-R is a 32-item instrument to measure patient satisfaction with acute migraine treatment comprising Efficacy, Functionality, Ease of Use, Cost and Tolerability scales. The PPMQ-R incorporates many inputs like those from patient groups, migraine-related literature, and clinical expert reviews [81]. PPMQ-R had a strong internal consistency (Cronbach's $\alpha$: 0.80–0.98) and test–retest reliability (intra-class correlation coefficient: 0.79–0.91) [82, 83]. PPMQ-R scale and Total scores (Efficacy, Functionality and Ease of use) demonstrated very good internal consistency reliability (a 0.84–0.99). Efficacy, Functionality and Total PPMQ-R scores showed large, reverse association with pain severity, number of migraine symptoms and work ability ($r = -0.62$ to $-0.75$; all $p < 0.0001$). All scales of PPMQ-R able to differentiate among migraine pain severity levels (all $p < 0.001$).

## 2.6   Conclusions

Measurement is a fundamental part of headache research, like many other topics. Researchers are often faced with the immense need to measure something that has not been approached previously or an efficacy of some new treatment modalities in headache disorders. Hence to minimize subjectivity, clinical scales and PROMs play an essential role for screening and assessing many aspects of headache such as severity of pain, associated features, disability, and burden of disease besides treatment outcomes. Therefore, many scales and PROM have been created in the last few decades as shortly summarized here.

We believe that these instruments may reduce time required for headache evaluation along with improving quantitative evaluation in follow-up visits. However, reliability and validity have a critical issue in using and evaluating these clinical scales. They may be subject to cultural diversity, because cultural differences and variations may affect a patient's assessment and understanding of each scale. Hence further research should be suggested to define if these scales are applicable to migraine patients who speak different languages. In the end of this chapter, we would like to encourage the readers and researchers to validate these scales that have not been studied in their own native languages to date.

# References


1. Stovner LJ, Hagen K, Jensen R, Katsarava Z, Lipton RB, Ai S, et al. The global burden of headache: a documentation of headache prevalence and disability worldwide. Cephalalgia. 2007;27:193–210.
2. World Health Organization and Lifting the Burden. Atlas of headache disorders and resources in the world. Geneva: WHO; 2011.
3. Food and Drug Administration (FDA), US Department of Health and Human Services (HHS). Patient-reported outcome measures; use in medical product development to support labeling claims. Guidance for Industry. https://www.fda.gov/regulatory-information/search-fda-guidance-documents/patient-reported-outcome-measures-use-medical-product-development-support-labeling-claims
4. Mokkink LB, Terwee CB, Patrick DL, Alonso J, Stratford PW, Knol DL, et al. The COSMIN study reached international status on taxonomy, terminology, and definitions of measurement properties for health-related patient reported outcomes. J Clin Epidemiol. 2010;63:737–45.
5. Terwee CB, Mokkink LB, Knol DL, Ostelo RWJG, Bouter LM, de Vet HCW. Rating the methodological quality in systematic reviews of studies on measurement properties. Qual Life Res. 2012;21:651–7.
6. Bossuyt PM, Reitsma JB, Bruns DE, Gatsonis CA, Glasziou PP, Irwig LM, et al. The STARD statement for reporting studies of diagnostic accuracy: explanation and elaboration. Ann Intern Med. 2003;138:1–12.
7. Page MJ, McKenzie JE, Bossuyt PM, Boutron I, Hoffmann TC, Mulrow CD, et al. The PRISMA 2020 statement: an updated guideline for reporting systematic reviews. BMJ. 2021;372:71.
8. von Elm E, Altman DG, Egger M, Pocock SJ, Gotzsche PC, Vandenbroucke JP. The Strengthening the Reporting of Observational Studies in Epidemiology (STROBE) statement: guidelines for reporting observational studies. Lancet. 2007;370(9596):1453–7.
9. Benchimol EI, Smeeth L, Guttmann A, Harron K, Moher D, Petersen I, RECORD Working Committee, et al. The REporting of studies Conducted using Observational Routinely-collected health Data (RECORD) statement. PLoS Med. 2015;12(10):e1001885.
10. Eigenbrodt AK, Asnina H, Khan S, Diener HC, Mitsikostas DD, Sinclair AJ, et al. Diagnosis and management of migraine in ten steps. Nat Rev Neurol. 2021;17:501–4.
11. Headache Classification Committee of the International Headache Society (IHS). The international classification of headache disorders, 3rd edition. Cephalalgia. 2018;38:1–211.
12. Dodick DW. Clinical clues and clinical rules: primary versus secondary headache. Adv Stud Med. 2003;3:550–5.
13. Lipton RB, Dodick D, Sadovsky R, Kolodner K, Endicott J, Hettiarachchi J, et al. A self-administered screener for migraine in primary care. The IDMigraine ™ validation study. Neurology. 2003;61:375–82.
14. Siva A, Zarifoglu M, Ertas M, Saip S, Karli HN, Baykan B, et al. Validity of the ID-Migraine screener in the workplace. Neurology. 2008;70(16):1337–45.
15. Ertaş M, Baykan B, Tuncel D, Gökçe M, Gökçay F, Sirin H, MIRA-3 Study Group, et al. A comparative ID migraine screener study in ophthalmology, ENT and neurology out-patient clinics. Cephalalgia. 2009;29(1):68–75. https://doi.org/10.1111/j.1468-2982.2008.01702.x.
16. Karli N, Ertas M, Baykan B, Uzunkaya O, Saip S, Zarifoglu M, MIRA Study Group, et al. The validation of ID Migraine screener in neurology outpatient clinics in Turkey. J Headache Pain. 2007;8(4):217–23.
17. Parakramaweera R, Evans RE, Schor LI, Pearson SM, Martines R, Cammarata, et al. A brief diagnostic screen for cluster headache: creation and initial validation of the Erwin Test for Cluster Headache. Cephalalgia. 2021;41(13):1298–309.
18. Maizels M, Burchette R. A rapid and sensitive paradigm for screening headache patients in primary care settings. Headache. 2003;43:441–50.
19. Maizels M, Houle T. Results of screening with the brief headache screen compared with a modified ID Migraine. Headache. 2008:385–94.

20. Láinez MJA, Domínguez M, Rejas J, Palacios G, Arriaza E, Garcia-Garcia M, et al. Development and validation of the Migraine Screen Questionnaire (MS-Q). Headache. 2005;45:1328–38.
21. Láinez MJ, Castillo J, Domínguez M, Palacios G, Díaz S, Rejas J. New uses of the Migraine Screen Questionnaire (MS-Q): validation in the Primary Care setting and ability to detect hidden migraine. MS-Q in Primary Care. BMC Neurol. 2010;10:39.
22. Maizels M, Wolfe WF. An expert system for headache diagnosis: the Computerized Headache Assessment Tool (CHAT). Headache. 2008;48:72–8.
23. Buse DC, Sollars CM, Steiner TJ, Jensen RH, Al Jumah MA, Lipton RB. Why HURT? A review of clinical instruments for headache management. Curr Pain Headache Rep. 2012;16:237–54.
24. Kosinski M, Bayliss MS, Bjorner JB, Ware JE, Garber WH, Batenhorst A, et al. A six-item short-form survey for measuring headache impact: the HIT-6. Qual Life Res. 2003;12:963–74.
25. Lipton RB, Varon SF, Grosberg B, McAllister PJ, Freitag F, Aurora SK, et al. OnabotulinumtoxinA improves quality of life and reduces impact of chronic migraine. Neurology. 2011;77:1465–72.
26. Yalinay PD, Bozdag M, Gunes M, Kosak S, Tasdelen B, Uluduz D, et al. Reliability and validity of Turkish version of Headache Impact Test (HIT-6) in patients with migraine. Arch Neuropsychiat. 2020;58(4):300–7.
27. Steiner DL, Norman GR, Cairney J. Health measurement scales: a practical guide to their development and use. 5th ed. Oxford: Oxford University Press; 2015.
28. de Vet H, Terwee CB, Mokkink LB, et al. Measurement in medicine. A practical guide. Cambridge: Cambridge University Press; 2011.
29. Coeytaux RR, Kaufman JS, Chao R, Mann JD, Devellis RF. Four methods of estimating the minimal important difference score were compared to establish a clinically significant change in Headache Impact Test. J Clin Epidemiol. 2006;59:374–80.
30. Smelt AF, Assendelt WF, Terwee CB, Ferrari MD, Blom JW. What is a clinically relevant change on the HIT-6 questionnaire? An estimation in a primary-care population of migraine patients. Cephalalgia. 2014;34:29–36.
31. Steiner TJ. The HALT and HART indices. J Headache Pain. 2007;8:22–5.
32. Steiner TJ, Lipton RB. Lifting the burden: the global campaign against headache. J Headache Pain. 2018;19:12.
33. Seleker HM, Gökmen G, Alvur TM, Steiner TJ. Productivity losses attributable to headache, and their attempted recovery, in a heavy-manufacturing workforce in Turkey: implications for employers and politicians. J Headache. 2015;16:96.
34. Jacobson GB, Ramadan RB, Aggarwal SK, Newman CW. The Henry Ford hospital disability inventory (HDI). Neurology. 1994;44:837–42.
35. Jacobson GB, Ramadan RB, Norris L, Newman CW. Headache Disability Inventory (HDI): short-term test-retest reliability and spouse perceptions. Headache. 1995;35:534–9.
36. Lipton RB, Stewart WF, Sawyer J, Edmeads JG. Clinical utility of an instrument assessing migraine disability: the Migraine Disability Assessment (MIDAS) questionnaire. Headache. 2001;41:854–61.
37. Stewart WF, Lipton RB, Simon D, et al. Reliability of an illness severity measure for headache in a population sample of migraine sufferers. Cephalalgia. 1998;18:44–51.
38. Kamm K, Straube A, Ruscheweyh R. Cluster Headache Impact Questionnaire (CHIQ) – a short measure of cluster headache related disability. J Headache Pain. 2022;23:37.
39. Andrée C, Vaillant M, Barré J, Katsarava Z, Lainez JM, Lair ML, et al. Development and validation of the EUROLIGHT questionnaire to evaluate the burden of primary headache disorders in Europe. Cephalalgia. 2010;30:1082–100. https://doi.org/10.1177/0333102409354323.
40. Steiner TJ, Stovner LR. Social impact of headache. Switzerland: Springer; 2019.
41. Vernon H, Lawson G. Development of the headache activities of daily living index: initial validity study. J Manip Physiol Ther. 2015;38:102–11.

42. Haywood KL, Mard TS, Potter R, Patel S, Matharu M, Underwood M. Assessing the impact of headaches and the outcomes of treatment: a systematic review of patient-reported outcome measures (PROMS). Cephalalgia. 2018;38:1374–86.

43. Niere K, Quin M. Development of a headache-specific disability questionnaire for patients attending physiotherapy. Man Ther. 2009;14:45–51.

44. Cramer JA, Silberstein SD, Winner P. Development and validation of the Headache Needs Assessment (HANA) survey. Headache. 2001;41:402–9.

45. El Hasnaoui A, Vray M, Richard A, MIGSEV Group, et al. Assessing the severity of migraine: development of the MIGSEV scale. Headache. 2003;43:628–35.

46. El Hasnaoui A, Vray M, Blin P, Nachit-Ouinekh F, Bureau F, HEMISPHERE study group. Assessment of migraine severity using the MIGSEV scale: relationship to migraine features and quality of life. Cephalalgia. 2004;24(4):262–70.

47. Stewart WF, Lipton RB, Kolodner K, Liberman J, Sawyer J. Reliability of the migraine disability assessment score in a population-based sample of headache sufferers. Cephalalgia. 1999;19:107–14.

48. Steward WF, Lipton RB, Dowson AJ, Sawyer J. Development and testing of the Migraine Disability Assessment (MIDAS) questionnaire to assess headache-related disability. Neurology. 2001;56:20–8.

49. Lipton RB, Desai P, Sapra S. How much change in headache-related disability is clinically meaningful? Estimating minimally important difference (MID) or change in MIDAS using data from the AMPP study. Headache. 2017;57:113–226. Abstract PF52–S113–226. Abstract PF52

50. Pathak DS, Chisolm DJ, Weis KA. Functional Assessment in Migraine (FAIM) questionnaire: development of an instrument based upon the WHO's International Classification of Functioning, Disability, and Health. Value Health. 2005;8:591–600.

51. Buse DC, Bigal MB, Rupnow M, Reed M, Serrano D, Lipton RB. Development and validation of the Migraine Interictal Burden Scale (MIBS): a self-administered instrument for measuring the burden of migraine between attacks (abstract S05.003). Neurology. 2007;68(suppl 1):A89.

52. Buse DC, Bigal M, Rupnow M, Leed M, Serrano D, Biondi DM, et al. The migraine interictal burden scale (MIBS): results of a population-based validation study. In: Headache, vol. 47; 2007. p. 778. Conference: 49th Annual Scientific Meeting of the American-Headache-Society.

53. Buse DC, Rupnow MF, Lipton RB. Assessing and managing all aspects of migraine: migraine attacks, migraine-related functional impairment, common comorbidities, and quality of life. Mayo Clin Proc. 2009;84:422–35.

54. Food Drug Administration (FDA). Guidance for industry patient-reported outcome measures: use in medical product development to support labeling claims. Fed Regist. 2009;74:65132–3.

55. Patrick DL, Burke LB, Gwaltney CJ, Leidy NK, Martin ML, Molsen E, et al. Content validity–establishing and reporting the evidence in newly developed patient-reported outcomes (PRO) instruments for medical product evaluation: ISPOR PRO good research practices task force report: part 1–eliciting concepts for a new PRO instrument. Value Health. 2011;14:967–77.

56. Patrick DL, Burke LB, Gwaltney CJ, Leidy NK, Martin ML, Molsen E, et al. Content validity–establishing and reporting the evidence in newly developed patient-reported outcomes (PRO) instruments for medical product evaluation: ISPOR PRO good research practices task force report: part 2–assessing respondent understanding. Value Health. 2011;14:978–88.

57. Hareendran A, Skalicky A, Mannix S, Lavoie S, Desai P, Bayliss M, et al. Development of a new tool for evaluating the benefit of preventive treatments for migraine on functional outcomes The Migraine Functional Impact Questionnaire (MFIQ). Headache. 2018;58:1612–28.

58. Tassorelli C, Diener HC, Dodick DW, Silberstein SD, Lipton RB, Ashina M, et al. Guidelines of the International Headache Society for controlled trials of preventive treatment of chronic migraine in adults. Cephalalgia. 2018;38:815–32.

59. Ware JE, Sherbourne CD. The MOS 36-Item Short Form Health Survey (SF-36). I: conceptual framework and item selection. Med Care. 1992;30(6):473–83.

60. Ware J, Kosinski M, Keller SD. A 12-item short-form health survey: construction of scales and preliminary tests of reliability and validity. Med Care. 1996;34:220–33.

61. Ware J, Kosinski M, Dewey J, Gondek B, Kosinski M, Ware J, et al. How to score and interpret single-item health status measures: a manual for users of the SF-8 health survey. Boston Quality Metric; 2001.

62. Solomon GD, Skobieranda FG, Gragg LA. Quality of life and well-being of headache patients: measurement by the Medical Outcomes Study instrument. Headache. 1993;33(7):351–8.
63. Osterhaus JT, Townsend RJ, Gandek B, Ware JE Jr. Measuring the functional status and well-being of patients with migraine headache. Headache. 1994;34(6):337–43.
64. Bussone G, Usai S, Gazzi L, Rigamonti A, Solari A, D' Amico D. Disability and quality of life in different primary headaches: results from Italian studies. Neurol Sci. 2004;25(suppl 3):105–7.
65. Magnusson JE, Riess CM, Becker WJ. Modification of the SF-36 for a headache population changes patient-reported health status. Headache. 2012;52:993–1004.
66. Lipton RB, Liberman JN, Kolodner KB, Bigal ME, Dowson A, Stewart WF. Migraine headache disability and health-related quality-of-life: a population-based case-control study from England. Cephalalgia. 2003;23(6):441–50.
67. The EuroQual Group. EuroQoL – a new facility for the measurement of health-related quality of life. Health Policy. 1990;16:199–208.
68. Xu R, Insigna RP, Golden W, Hu XL. EuroQoL (EQ-5D) health utility scores for patients with migraine. Qual Life Res. 2011;20(4):601–8.
69. Jhidran P, Osterhaus JT, Miller DW, Lee JT, Kirchdoerfer L. Development and validation of the migraine-specific quality of life questionnaire. Headache. 1998;38:295–302.
70. Martin BC, Pathak DS, Sharfman MI, Adelman JU, Taylor F, Kwong WJ, et al. Validity and reliability of the migraine-specific quality of life questionnaire (MSQ version 2.1). Headache. 2000;40:204–15.
71. Cole JC, Lin P, Rupnow MF. Minimal important differences in the Migraine-Specific Quality of Life Questionnaire (MSQ) version 2.1. Cephalalgia. 2009;29:1180–7.
72. Buse DC, Lipton RB, Hallström Y, Reuter U, Tepper SJ, et al. Migraine-related disability, impact, and health-related quality of life among patients with episodic migraine receiving preventive treatment with Erenumab. Cephalalgia. 2018;38:1622–31.
73. Rendas-Baum R, Bloudel LM, Maglinte GA, Varon SF. The psychometric properties of the Migraine-Specific Quality of Life Questionnaire version 2.1 (MSQ) in chronic migraine patients. Qual Life Res. 2013;22:1123–33.
74. Conn CD, Fehnel SE, Davis KH, Runken MC, Beach ME, Cady RK. The development of a survey to measure completeness of response to migraine therapy. Headache. 2012;52:550–72.
75. Dowson AJ, Tepper SJ, Baos V, Baudet F, D'Amico D, Kilminster S. Identifying patients who require a change in their current acute migraine treatment: the Migraine Assessment of Current Therapy (migraine-ACT) questionnaire. Curr Med Res Opin. 2004;20:1125–35.
76. Chatterton ML, Lofland JH, Shechter A, Curtice WS, Hu HX, Lenow J, et al. Reliability and validity of migraine therapy assessment questionnaire. Headache. 2002;42:106–1015.
77. Landis JR, Koch GG. The measurement of observer agreement for categorical data. Biometrics. 1977;33:159.
78. Ware JE Jr, Bjorner JB, Kosinski M. Practical implications of item response theory and computerized adaptive testing: a brief summary of ongoing studies of widely used headache impact scales [comment]. Med Care. 2000;38(9 suppl):II73–82.
79. Lipton RB, Kolodner K, Bigal ME, Valade D, Lainez MJA, Pascual J, et al. Validity and reliability of migraine-treatment optimization questionnaire. Cephalalgia. 2009;29:751–9.
80. Patrick DL, Martin ML, Bushnell DM, Pesa J. Measuring satisfaction with migraine treatment: expectations, importance, outcomes, and global ratings. Clin Ther. 2003;25:2920–35.
81. Davis KH, Black L, Sleath B. Validation of the patient perception of migraine questionnaire. Value Health. 2002;5:421–9.
82. Revicki DA, Kimel M, Beusterien K, Kwong JW, Varner JA, Amer MH, et al. Validation of the revised patient perception of migraine questionnaire: measuring satisfaction with acute migraine treatment. Headache. 2006;46:240–52.
83. Kimel M, Hsieh R, McCormack J, Burch SP, Revicki DA. Validation of the revised Patient Perception of Migraine Questionnaire (PPMQ-R): measuring satisfaction with acute migraine treatment in clinical trials. Cephalalgia. 2008;28:510–23.

# Chapter 3
# Reliability and Validity of Clinical Scales Measurement

Hüseyin Selvi and Aynur Özge

## 3.1 Introduction

Any attempt at carrying a significantly subjective sensation over into an entirely objective context will require a significant amount of effort and mastery. A further attempt at transforming this objective context into a series of indicators that would bring different individuals to the same conclusion, in turn, requires an even higher level of mastery and craft. In this part, we will check over the processes involved in the development of a scale, as well as the validity and reliability of clinical scales to be employed in the diagnosis and treatment of headaches. We will focus on distinct elements of the matter that will offer guidance to clinicians by keeping the technical aspects to the possible minimum. The ability of any tool developed to measure a subjective variable for clinical purposes to produce on-point decisions is essential for accuracy in diagnosis, patient referral, and treatment processes.

Reaching right decisions, however, is not as difficult as commonly believed. The toolbox required for this purpose must consist of a qualified measurement procedure and an assessment process employing a criterion/a set of criteria that is fit for purpose. Qualified measurement procedures, in turn, can only be developed with the use of measurement tools with established reliability and validity.

H. Selvi
Associated Professor of Medical Education Department, Mersin University Medical School, Mersin, Turkey

A. Özge (✉)
Department of Neurology, Mersin University Medical School, Mersin, Turkey



P. Yalınay Dikmen, A. Özge (eds.), *Clinical Scales for Headache Disorders*, Headache, https://doi.org/10.1007/978-3-031-25938-8_3

## 3.2   Developing a Clinical Scale

Decisions to be made by physicians about patients can directly affect patient health and life. In this process, patients may not only regain their health, but also wait for a long time to regain their health and miss the chance of early diagnosis/treatment, which is important for the treatment of some diseases. For this reason, it is extremely important for the health and life of the patients that physicians make accurate decisions in the diagnosis and treatment processes.

The more reliable and valid information about the patient and the disease is in front of the physician, the healthier the diagnosis and treatment process will be. For this reason, it is extremely important for the diagnosis and treatment processes to provide reliable and valid information to the physicians that will be the basis for making accurate decisions about the patient and the disease.

Providing this information is possible with clinical scales with proven reliability and validity. The development processes of clinical scales are directly related to the variable to be measured from the patient. As a matter of fact, the development processes of clinical scales are different in cases where a directly observable variable such as the patient's blood pressure, body temperature, and blood gas will be measured; It works differently in situations where a variable that cannot be directly observed, such as anxiety and depression, will be measured. The main purpose here is to measure the variable to be measured from the patient without mixing with other features (validity) and without error (reliability). These concepts will be explained in more detail in the following sections.

## 3.3   Measurement of a Clinical Scale

### 3.3.1   Basic Concept

In the simplest terms, the concept of measurement can be defined as the quantification of qualities. Here, 'quality' refers to a property of interest for the researcher, while 'quantification' is the process of matching the extent to which the property of interest is present in a variable with numbers, symbols, adjectives, or signs [1–3]. Measurement procedures employed in clinical contexts entail the use of measurement tools devised specifically for intended purposes.

A measurement procedure involving the use of a scale can be conducted in one of two forms, i.e., direct and indirect measurement and at one of four levels, namely nominal, ordinal, equal interval, and ratio [4, 5].

In *direct measurement*, the property measured will be similar to/the same as the property of the scale employed to measure that specific property. In other words, the property of interest is measured in a variable by way of direct observation and without any need for an additional property. Examples of direct measurements include procedures to determine the number of patients in the polyclinic waiting list, to establish the duration of pain in a headache patient, and to find out the length of hospitalisation of inpatients.

On the other hand, *indirect measurement* is used when the measured property differs from the property targeted by the tool employed for its measurement. In other words, when a property of a variable does not lend itself to direct observation, it is instead established through the measurement of another property of the same variable that can be observed directly and is considered/known to be associated with that property. Examples of this type of measurement include measurements based on reactions to scale items as is the case in the measurement of intelligence, the determination of pain severity in a headache patient, and the identification of state-trait anxiety level.

Another type of measurement considered in the category of indirect measurements is *derived measurement.* Derived measurement represents a measurement process carried out through mathematical relations based on measurements taken on a set of different properties without any measurement conducted on the variable. Examples of this type of measurement include the calculation of medical dosage through assessments of such variables as age, weight, and height, etc.

In *nominal measurement level*, individuals are divided into categories on the basis of whether they possess the property of interest or not. Measurements collected on a nominal level are more compatible with counting exercises and as such, they lend themselves to only a limited number of statistical analyses. An example of nominal measurement may be the placement of a sign on the door of a room housing in patients with balance problems in order to separate them from those without.

In *ordinal measurement level*, individuals are placed in a rough order in line with whether they possess the property of interest or not. An example of ordinal measurement may be found in the ordinal measurement undertaken to put patients visiting an emergency service by clinical status.

In *equal-interval measurement level*, individuals are placed on a scale featuring a fixed unit that remains constant between measurements and a starting point (zero point) in line with the extent to which they possess the property of interest. The starting point mentioned here (zero point) does not indicate a true absence. As it is possible to aggregate measurements taken on an equal-interval scale, they lend themselves to a large number of statistical analyses including calculations of arithmetic average, standard deviation, normal distribution, variance, inter-group differences, and correlation. Measurements taken at intervals on a scale such as the visual analogue scale of pain intensity may be considered as an example of equal-interval measurement.

Finally, in *ratio measurement level*, variables are placed on a scale featuring a fixed unit that remains constant between measurements and a starting point (zero point) in line with the extent to which they possess the property of interest as is the case in equal-interval measurement. However, the starting point specified here (zero point) does represent a true absence. As it is also possible to aggregate measurements taken on a ratio scale in a manner similar to the equal-interval scale, they lend themselves to a large number of statistical analyses including calculations of arithmetic average, standard deviation, normal distribution, variance, inter-group differences, and correlation. An example of this type of measurement may be the ratio measurement of heart rate variability during pain.

### 3.3.2 Measurement Tools

Measurement tools are classified and named in line with the purposes for which they have been developed. The levels of measurement governing the measures taken on measurement tools also depend on the qualification of the tool used for measurement. It is, therefore, possible to collect data at different measurement levels through the combined use of diverse measurement tools. For example, a survey may pose the question 'What is your gender?' to collect nominal data and allow for some limited statistical analyses based on this data set, whereas the same survey may also ask 'How old are you?' as a means to collecting ratio data and making it possible for a researcher to conduct more advanced statistical analyses based on the resulting data set.

Measurement tools can be divided into two types: measurement tools assessing **maximum performance** by taking individuals through a process where they must do their best and, in general, compete with others or themselves in doing so and measurement tools measuring **typical behaviours** exhibited by individuals without any additional effort in their own environment. In this context, tests are employed for the measurement of maximum performance, while typical behaviours are measured on scales [6].

## 3.4   Assessment

### 3.4.1 Basic Concept

Although clinical measurement tools are put in use with established reliability and validity, the measurements taken on these tools do not mean anything by themselves [7]. In other words, an individual scoring 75 on a clinical scale is not an indication of whether they have a clinical problem or not. A criterion score will be needed to reach such an indication. The process through which an individual's score is compared to a reference score(s) to guide a decision on their clinical status is called an **assessment** [6]. Therefore, a measurement result must be benchmarked with a reference score before a decision may be made as to whether an individual is anxious/not anxious, ill/not ill or in mild pain/in severe pain, etc. through the use of a scale regardless of the purpose for which it has been developed [7]. An assessment may employ one of four different references:

Domain-referenced assessment
Cut-off score-based assessment
Rank-based assessment
Norm-referenced assessment

### 3.4.2   Domain-Referenced Assessment

When an individual scores 150 on a scale, this result does not mean anything by itself. However, if the maximum possible score on this scale were known at least, the individual's score of 150 on the scale could become more meaningful. For example, if the maximum possible score on this scale is 150, it will be possible to indicate that the individual possesses the property measured by the scale at the maximum level. If, however, the maximum possible score on this scale is 600, it will be possible to conclude that the individual possesses only 25% of the property measured by the scale. Therefore, the knowledge of the maximum score possible on a scale will add meaning to an individual's score and the maximum score possible on a scale may be taken as a reference as it represents 100% of the property of interest for the scale [6, 7].

### 3.4.3   Cut-Off Score-Based Assessment

A cut-off score can be used as a reference to add meaning to a scale score. The cut-off score mentioned here can be defined as the level of minimum acceptable performance. For example, individuals scoring 60 or higher in an anxiety scale may be considered to have anxiety, while those scoring lower than 60 may be described as anxiety-free. The score of 60 here is the cut-off score, which refers to the threshold value that separates individuals with anxiety from those without. In this context, it is possible to identify a single cut-off score to assess overall level of anxiety or multiple cut-off scores to establish different levels of anxiety. A range of methods have been developed in the literature to determine such cut-off scores for measurement tools including Angoff, Ebel, and Nedelsky [8]. The choice of these methods depend on the type of measurement tool and scoring to be applied; however, they are typically based on the averaging of scale score estimates of patients at maximum performance from (*at least five and ideally ten or more*) specialised physicians with a good command of the illness concerned and of relevant patients.

### 3.4.4  Rank-Based Assessment

This type of assessment focuses on the rank which an individual is placed at by reason of their score on a scale. In other words, the assessment is based on the ranking of an individual among all responding individuals with their score rather than their actual score on the scale. For example, if ten individuals take a stress test and the aim is to identify three individuals with the lowest levels of stress among them, the responding individuals will be ranked from the lowest to the highest with their scale scores, allowing for the identification of three top-ranking individuals. This type of assessment is considered when there is a quota for the number of persons to be identified on a scale [6].

### 3.4.5  Norm-Referenced Assessment

In this type of assessment, the scale score of an individual is provided with a meaning through the use of the arithmetic average and standard deviation identified for the entire group of respondents. To this end, the points scored by an individual on a scale is converted into a standard score, which is, in turn, employed to establish the number of standard deviations that make up the distance between the individual's score and the average score of their own group. In addition, in cases where the measured property varies in proportion with another variable such as age or gender, this assessment allows for this other variable to be taken into account. For instance, let's imagine the height of a person measured at 60 cm; age will be a significant variable in the interpretation of this measurement result. In fact, a height of 60 cm will mean one thing for a 10-year-old and another for a 20-year-old. In other words, it is possible to add meaning to the height measurement of an individual also in the context of their other properties including age, gender, and race [9].

## 3.5  Qualification Requirements for Clinical Measurement Tools

There are two fundamental qualities any measurement tool must satisfy in order for the data obtained through its use to be used as a basis for on-point decisions, namely reliability and validity. Finally, errors have to taken account at this step.

### 3.5.1  Reliability

The reliability of a scale is expressed as its ability to provide error-free measurements.

The literature defines reliability as;

- 'Freedom from random errors in measurement results [7],
- Ratio of true score variance to the total variance of observed scores [10],
- Ability of a measurement tool to offer the same result under the same conditions' [11].

In short, reliability refers to the sensitivity, stability, and consistency of measurements obtained from a measurement tool.

In this context, *sensitivity* concerns the unit of a given scale. Regardless of the specific measurement tool used, reliability increases as the unit gets smaller [7]. For example, weighing a new-born in grams will result in more measurements than weighing it in kilograms. Similarly, using milligrams instead of grams while preparing medication for a patient will result in a more sensitive and precise mixing ratio.

*Stability* pertains to the scale being able to provide the same result between repeated applications. Here, the measured property must remain the same between the initial and repeated applications. For example, let's measure a patient's body temperature twice in a row. Unless there has been a change in the patient's body temperature after the initial measurement, any difference between the two consecutive measurements will indicate that the thermometer used has an error in measurement. Similarly, when measuring the weight of an infant twice in a row at a 30-s interval, any variation between the two measurements will make us think of a possible error in the scales used. The 'test-retest'' method is used to determine the stability reliability of a scale [6, 7].

*Consistency* concerns the general agreement between the items (questions) on a scale and the scale as a whole. An example of consistency reliability may be an intelligence test developed to measure the intelligence of individuals featuring questions measuring intelligence in all of its items or a weighing device offering accurate measurements of different weights. The consistency reliability of a scale is determined with such methods as KR-20 and KR-21 for dichotomously scores scales (0–1) or with Cronbach alpha, Rulon, and Guttman, etc. for polytomous scores scales [12, 13].

In summary, reliability can be defined as the level of freedom from error and accuracy in measurement results. The mathematical expression of reliability is as given in Eq. (3.1).

$$r_{xx} = \frac{True\,Score}{Observed\,Score} \tag{3.1}$$

A closer look at Eq. (3.1) shows that the closer observed score is to true score, the closer the reliability coefficient will be to 1.00 and in turn, the reliability coefficient will move towards 0.00 as observed score moves away from true score. This equation tells us that reliability is a measurement of freedom from error. In other words, reliability does not indicate the magnitude of error that gets into measurement results. Measurement results are considered to be reliable with the reliability coefficient moving closer to 1.00 and to be unreliable as it gets closer to 0.00. A reliability value of 0.70 or higher is needed for a measurement tool to offer reliable measurements [14].

### 3.5.1.1 Methods to Assess Reliability in Clinical Scales

There are a range of methods employed to calculate the reliability of clinical scales and the choice depends on the theory applied, the type of error in measurement results, and the distinct quality to be assessed, i.e. sensitivity, consistency, or stability.

This part of the book will consider two categories of methods used to determine reliability in scales in line with the classical test theory, namely methods based on multiple applications and methods based on a single application.

## 3.5.2 Validity

The validity of a scale relates to the extent to which it serves its intended purpose. In the literature, validity is defined as 'the ability of a scale to measure the property it intends to measure without confounding it with any other properties' [3]. Studies that look into the validity of scales seek answers to the question 'What does the scale measure and how good is it at doing that?' [2].

Here, the concept of validity will be considered under two headings, namely measurement validity where the focus is on the validity of scales, and decision validity where the point in question concerns the accuracy of decisions rendered with respect to individuals on the basis of scores obtained from such scales.

### 3.5.2.1 Measurement Validity

Measurement validity is defined as the degree to which a scale serves its intended purpose. In other words, it can be specified as a scale actually measuring what it intends to measure. A scale must fulfil the requirements of content validity, criterion-related validity, and construct validity in order to be considered as serving its intended purpose [6, 15].

Content Validity

Content validity is concerned with the extent to which a scale is able to offer an accurate reflection of the property it intends to measure. If we consider the indicative behaviours of the property to be measured as a universe, content validity can be explained as the degree to which a scale is able to reflect this universe [1].

The first step to assessing and securing content validity is to offer a good explanation of what the measured property is and what it is not. In other words, content validity must be based on a precise delineation of the property to be measured. This delineation, in turn, requires discussions on the measured property with experts with a good level of familiarity with the property in question, a literature review on the measured property, and an examination of the other scales developed for similar purposes. There are a number of methods developed in the literature to secure content validity. Common examples include the Davis technique and Lawshe's technique. As these techniques are put to use in the development of scales, they will not be considered in detail here [16–18].

Criterion-Related Validity

Criterion-related validity concerns the ability of a scale to produce similar measurements to those of another, validated scale developed for a similar purpose. For an assessment of criterion-related validity, another scale developed for a similar purpose is to be identified as the gold standard; the two scales are applied to the same group of individuals and the scores obtained are then used to calculate inter-score correlation. The resulting correlation value will offer an idea about the criterion-related validity of the scale [18].

Criterion-related validity is referred to as concurrent validity when the scores to be considered as the gold standard are already available or as predictive validity when such scores are to be obtained at a later time [18].

Construct Validity

Clinical scales are usually intended to measure psychological variables. Psychological variables, however, cannot be observed directly. Therefore, targeted scales are developed for the measurement of these variables that don't lend themselves to direct observation. In turn, the responses of patients or physicians to the items posed to them in such scales are employed to establish the relevant psychological construct [19].

Construct validity is the type of validity where the aim is to establish whether the psychological construct a clinical scale intends to measure is, in fact, the structure that is being measured by the scale. In other words, construct validity determines whether a scale does practically measure the structure it aims to measure in theory. To this end, examinations are required on the agreement among the responses given by individuals to scale items, the individual factors in the scale, the agreement among factors and between factors and their sub-items, and the variance ratio expressed by the scale, etc. The literature offers statistical analyses developed for this purpose. However, the most common analysis used in studies of construct validity is the factor analysis. Factor analysis is considered in two parts, namely exploratory factor analysis that tries to establish the theoretical construct a scale intends to measure and confirmatory factor analysis that tries to confirm whether the theoretical construct established by a scale is, in fact, the construct originally intended to be measured [20]. As these analyses are put to use in the development of scales, they will not be considered in detail here.

### 3.5.2.2 Decision Validity

Decision validity pertains to the accuracy of decisions made on the basis of scores obtained on a scale. In fact, even when a measurement tool with established reliability and validity is used, the use of a wrong cut-off score may result in a wrong decision being made for a patient on the basis of the scores obtained from the tool. Therefore, the validity of the cut-off score used for a scale is at least as important as the reliability and validity of the scale itself and decision validity must be considered in all studies looking into the validity of clinical scales [6]. There are many methods developed in the literature to stablish cut-off scores and assess decision validity. The most common methods developed to determine cut-off scores include Angoff, Ebel, Nedelsky, Jaeger, and Beuk, etc. and methods employed commonly to assess classification and ordinal consistencies of cut-off scores include the double-consistency index proposed by Erkus (2000) $(P_{CT})$ (Eq. (3.2)) and z index proposed by Subkoviak (1988) (Eq. (3.3)) [12, 21].

$$P_{CT} = 1 - \left[ \frac{\left( f_{ut} - f_{uc} \right) + \left( f_{at} - f_{ac} \right)}{N_{u+a}} \right] \tag{3.2}$$

$f_{ut}$ = number of diagnosed individuals from the top 27% as per the cut-off score
$f_{uc}$ = number of non-diagnosed individuals from the top 27% as per the cut-off score
$f_{at}$ = number of diagnosed individuals from the bottom 27% as per the cut-off score
$f_{ac}$ = number of non-diagnosed individuals from the bottom 27% as per the cut-off score
$N_{u+a}$ = number of individuals in bottom and top groups

$$IzI = \frac{\left( cutoff\ score - 0.5 - \text{Mean} \right)}{Std.d} \tag{3.3}$$

The values calculated through Eqs. (3.2) and (3.3) vary between 0.00 and 1.00. The closer the value is to 0.00 the less consistent the decisions made on the basis of the results will be and the closer it is to 1.00 the more consistent they will be. It is reported that this value must be 0.85 or higher for a scale to achieve decision validity [12, 21].

### 3.5.2.3  A Rundown on Reliability and Validity in Clinical Scales

- If a measurement tool is valid, it is definitely reliable at the same time.
- A reliable measurement tool may not be valid.
- The reliability of a measurement tool will limit its validity.
- Reliability is necessary, but not sufficient for validity.
- Reliability and validity are a matter of grading and therefore, it is not right to express them in absolute terms of presence or absence.
- The established reliability and validity of a scale do not guarantee that it will be a good basis for accurate decision-making; decision validity should be examined separately.

## *3.5.3  Error in Measurement*

Errors in measurement results may come from many sources including the environment, the scale, the person applying the scale, or the person that is assessed through the scale. Errors in measurement are divided into three categories depending on the magnitude and direction of error and whether the error comes from a known or unknown source [14].

***Constant error***  happens when the source, direction, and magnitude of an error in measurement results can be known. A constant error means that the error observed in measurement results is in the same direction and of the same magnitude. An example of a constant error would be a weighing device adding 50 g to every measurement. This type of errors affects the validity rather than reliability of scales.

***Systematic error***  is the type of error where, similar to a constant error, the source, direction, and magnitude of an error in measurement results can be known. However, the error observed in measurement results varies between measurements and as such, is not fixed. It either increases or decreases between measurements. An example of a systematic error would be a weighing device adding 10% to every measurement. Using this weighing device, 100 g would be measured as 110 and 150 g as 165 g, meaning that the magnitude of the error would be 10 g in one measurement and 15 g in another. As can be seen in this example, the direction, magnitude, and source of the error are known. Systematic errors affect the validity rather than reliability of scales in a manner similar to constant error.

***Random error***  happens when the source, direction, and magnitude of an error in measurement results cannot be known. There may be an error in measurement associated with a number of sources including the environment, chance success, the person undertaking the measurement, and the person being measured. Therefore, the magnitude of error in measurement results may increase or decrease irregularly.

An example of a random error would be a weighing device adding 10 g to one measurement and taking out 25 g from another. Random errors affect the reliability of scales.

### 3.5.3.1 Standard Error of Measurement

The values calculated with the abovementioned methods of assessing reliability range between 0.00 and 1.00. The closer this value is to 1.00 the more reliable the scores obtained on a scale and the closer it is to 0.00 the less reliable the scores. This value must be 0.70 or higher for a scale to be considered reliable.

Reliability is an indication of freedom from error in measurement results. Cases where there is an error observed in measurement results, however, call for the calculation of the standard error of measurement in order to establish the magnitude of the error in question. The reliability value calculated for a scale does vary due to the level of heterogeneity in its group of subjects, while such variation is not observed in the calculation of the standard error of measurement. As such, the standard error of measurement is a better tool in interpreting individual scores [3]. The standard error of measurement can be calculated with Eq. (3.4).

$$Se = Sx\sqrt{1 - r_x} \tag{3.4}$$

$Se$ = Standard error of measurement.
$Sx$ = Standard deviation of scale.
$r_x$ = Reliability coefficient of scale.

## 3.6 Reliability Methods for Clinical Scales

### 3.6.1 Method for Multiple Applications

### 3.6.1.1 Alternate Form Method

When an alternative (equivalent) is available to the scale in use, applying both scales to the same individuals and calculating the correlation between the resulting scores will offer an idea about the reliability of the original scale. The correlation value calculated here is called the _equivalence coefficient_. For two scales to be considered equivalent-parallel, they must be equal in terms of their average, variance, and covariance. It is extremely difficult, however, to find two scales that meet this requirement [7].

### 3.6.1.2 Test-Retest Method

This method is based on the repeated application of a single scale to the same group of individuals and under the same conditions but at different times. The correlation coefficient calculated between the scores obtained from the two applications will inform an assessor about the reliability of the scale. The correlation value here is referred to as the _coefficient of stability_ [16]. When one scale is applied to the same individuals twice, the exact time interval between the two applications depends on the nature of the variable being measured. The shorter this time interval is, the more likely the individuals will be to remember and as such, repeat their initial response at the second application. When there is a longer time interval between the applications, however, the resulting correlation coefficient will be lower due to the inevitable change in the behaviour being measured itself. Therefore, the time interval between the two applications should be long enough to prevent individuals from remembering their initial response, but short enough to make sure that the variable of interest remains constant between the applications [22].

## 3.6.2 Methods Based on a Single Application

Reliability assessment methods based on a single application entail the one-time application of a scale to a group of individuals and the examination of the consistency among scale items. The resulting value is referred to as the _coefficient of internal consistency_ [13, 14, 22].

### 3.6.2.1 Split-Half Method

The Conventional Method and Spearman-Brown Prophecy

In the conventional method of assessing reliability, a scale is to be split into two halves containing an equal number of items. In other words, a scale of 20 items will be split into two halves of ten items each. Then, the two halves are applied to the same group of individuals and a calculation is made to determine the correlation value between the scores. The correlation value, in turn, offers an idea about the reliability of the scale. However, the reliability value calculated in this way will only establish reliability for half of the scale only. Therefore, the calculated value of reliability should be extrapolated to the entire scale by using the formula given in Eq. (3.5). This equation is known in the literature as Spearman-Brown prophecy formula [13, 14].

$$r_{ho} = \frac{2r_{ab}}{1+r_{ab}} \tag{3.5}$$

$r_{ab}$ = _correlation between the first and second halves_
$r_{total}$ = _full-test reliability_

### 3.6.2.2   Rulon Method

Rulon method to determine reliability entails a scale being split into equal halves by the number of items in a manner similar to the conventional method. The two halves are applied to the same group of individuals followed by a calculation of the difference between the scores. The variance of difference and the variance of sum scores are then put into Eq. (3.6) to calculate the reliability value. Using the Spearman-Brown correction is not necessary for this method [7].

$$r_{rulon} = 1 - \left( \frac{S_f^2}{S_X^2} \right) \tag{3.6}$$

$S_f^2$ = *variance of the difference between the first and second halves*
$S_X^2$ = *variance of sum scores*

### 3.6.2.3   Guttman's Method

Guttman's method was derived from the Rulon method. In this method, the items on a scale are divided into two equal halves. Each half is applied to the same group of individuals and the variance values of the resulting scores and the total score are calculated separately. Then, Eq. (3.7) is used to calculate the reliability value through these variance values [7].

$$r_{guttman} = 2 \left[ 1 - \left( \frac{S_a^2 + S_b^2}{S_X^2} \right) \right] \tag{3.7}$$

$S_a^2$ = *variance of the first half*
$S_b^2$ = *variance of the second half*
$S_X^2$ = *variance of sum scores*

### 3.6.3   *Methods Based on Inter-item Covariance*

### 3.6.3.1   Kuder-Richardson Method (KR-20)

The KR-20 method to assess reliability is used for the calculation of the reliability of dichotomously scores scales in terms of internal consistency. Equation (3.8) can be used to calculate KR-20 [14].

$$KR-20 = \frac{K}{K-1} \left( 1 - \frac{\sum_{i=1}^{k} p * q}{S_x^2} \right) \tag{3.8}$$

$K$ = *number of scale items*
$p$ = *item-level proportion-correct score*
$q$ = *item-level proportion-incorrect score*
$S^2_X$ = *variance of sum scores*

### 3.6.3.2 Cronbach's Alpha Method

Cronbach's Alpha method of assessing reliability is used for the calculation of the reliability of polytomous scores scales in terms of internal consistency. Likert scales are an example of scales where this method may be employed to determine reliability. The Cronbach's Alpha reliability value can be calculated by using Eq. (3.9) [14, 15].

$$Cronbach\ Alpha = \frac{K}{K-1}\left(1 - \frac{\sum_{i=1}^{k} S_i^2}{S_x^2}\right) \tag{3.9}$$

$K$ = *number of scale items*
$p$ = *item-level proportion-correct score*
$q$ = *item-level proportion-incorrect score*
$S_i^2$ = *variance of items*
$S^2_X$ = *variance of sum scores*

## 3.7 Conclusions

- Any attempt at carrying an objectively subjective sensation over into an entirely objective context requires the use of scales that will offer cross-sectional and longitudinal assessments of every component of pain.
- The development of any such scale should consider the exact variable to be measured, the nature of the variable in question, and factors relating to the person undertaking the measurement altogether.
- The validity and reliability of each scale developed as such should be calculated as instructed.
- Analyses at every stage should also consider calculations of errors relating to patients and physicians.

## References

1. Murphy KR, Davidshofer CO. Psychological testing: principles and applications. Upper Saddle River, NJ: Prentice Hall; 2005.
2. Anastasi A, Urbina S. Psychological testing. Prentice Hall/Pearson Education; 1997.

3. Aiken LR. Psychological testing and assessment. Boston: Allyn and Bacon; 2000.
4. Dybkaer R, Jørgensen K. Measurement, value, and scale. Scand J Clin Lab Invest Suppl. 1989;194:69–76.
5. Tandy RD. Technical note: the initial stages of statistical data analysis. J Athl Train. 1998;33(1):69–71.
6. Erkus A, Selvi H. Measurement and scale development in psychology III-scale adaptation and norm development. Ankara: Pegem Akademi; 2021.
7. Lord FM, Novick MR. Statistical theories of mental test scores. Menlo Park: Addison-Wesley; 1968.
8. Yudkowsky R, Downing SM, Wirth S. Simpler standards for local performance examinations: the Yes/No Angoff and whole-test Ebel. Teach Learn Med. 2008;20(3):212–7. https://doi.org/10.1080/10401330802199450.
9. Royal KD, Guskey TR. On the appropriateness of norm- and criterion-referenced assessments in medical education. Ear Nose Throat J. 2015;94(7):252–4. https://doi.org/10.1177/014556131509400703.
10. Baykul Y. Productivity and evaluation in education. Education. 1992;113(2):307–11.
11. Erkuş A. A new index proposal: double consistency index. Turk J Psychol. 2000;15(46):63–71.
12. Uzun N, Alıcı D, Aktaş M. Reliability of the analytic rubric and checklist for the assessment of story writing skills: G and decision study in generalizability theory. Eurasian J Educ Res. 2019;8(1):169–80.
13. Crocker L, Algina J. Introduction to classical and modern test theory. Orlando, FL: Holt, Rinehart and Winston; 1986.
14. Magnusson D. Test theory. Boston: Addison-Wesley; 1967.
15. Haidari S, Uzun N. Content validity and confirmatory factor analysis of cooperative learning attitude scale (CLAS) for the EFL students. Int J Soc Sci Educ Res. 2015;5(1):418–33.
16. Polit DF, Beck CT, Owen SV. Is the CVI an acceptable indicator of content validity? Appraisal and recommendations. Res Nurs Health. 2007;30(4):459–67. https://doi.org/10.1002/nur.20199.
17. Esquivel Garzón N, Díaz Heredia LP. Validity and reliability of the treatment adherence questionnaire for patients with hypertension. Investig Educ Enferm. 2019;37(3):e09. https://doi.org/10.17533/udea.iee.v37n3e09.
18. Van Iddekinge CH, Roth PL, Raymark PH, Odle-Dusseau HN. The criterion-related validity of integrity tests: an updated meta-analysis. J Appl Psychol. 2012;97(3):499–530. https://doi.org/10.1037/a0021196.
19. Alıcı D. Developing the attitudes towards school scale: reliability and validity study. Educ Sci. 2013;38(1):318–31.
20. Thompson B. Exploratory and confirmatory factor analysis: understanding concepts and applications. Washington, DC; 2004.
21. Subkoviak MJ. A practitioner's guide to computation and interpretation of reliability indices for mastery tests. J Educ Meas. 1988;25(1):47–55.
22. Aktaş M, Alıcı D. Developing the attitude scale towards measurement and evaluation lesson in education. J Qafqaz Univ. 2012;33(1):66–73.

# Chapter 4
# Patient Reported Outcome Measures (PROMs) in Migraine and Headache

Dawn C. Buse and Richard B. Lipton

## 4.1 Introduction

Patient reported outcome measures (PROMs) are important for a variety of research and clinical purposes. PROMs gather data directly from people living with a disease reflecting some aspect of their disease experience. For conditions like migraine, where objective indicators of illness severity and treatment benefits are not available, PROMs provide crucial information on disease burden and therapeutic benefit. In this chapter we will provide an overview of PROM definitions, development and validation processes, interpretation, and use in both migraine clinical trials and clinical care.

Patient reported outcome measures (PROMs) are used in clinical trials to measure the benefits of treatment for outcomes best reported by patients. Regulatory agencies, such as the Food and Drug Administration (FDA) in the US and the European Medicines Agency (EMA) in the European Union, are responsible for ensuring the safety, efficacy, and security of drugs, biological products, and medical devices. Randomized controlled trials (RCTs) are essential to the generation of

Sponsorship: This chapter was supported by the Food and Drug Administration (FDA) of the U.S. Department of Health and Human Services (HHS) as part of a financial assistance award (UG3FD006795) totaling $1,599,834 with 100% funded by FDA/HHS. The contents are those of the authors and do not necessarily represent the official views of, nor an endorsement, by FDA/HHS, or the U.S. Government

D. C. Buse (✉)
Department of Neurology, Albert Einstein College of Medicine, Bronx, NY, USA
e-mail: dawnbuse@gmail.com

R. B. Lipton
Edwin S. Lowe Professor and Vice Chair of Neurology, Professor of Epidemiology and Population Health, Professor of Psychiatry and Behavioral Science, Albert Einstein College of Medicine, Montefiore Headache Center, Bronx, NY, USA
e-mail: richard.lipton@einstein.yu.edu



P. Yalınay Dikmen, A. Özge (eds.), *Clinical Scales for Headache Disorders*, Headache, https://doi.org/10.1007/978-3-031-25938-8_4

evidence on the efficacy, safety, and tolerability of treatments. RCTs specify primary and secondary endpoints based on the outcomes that are most salient for the most important stakeholders. In clinical trials, operationally defined endpoints examined by a limited number of statistical tests can determine whether treatment works to a statistically significant degree in producing prespecified outcomes. Primary endpoints in Phase III trials are often intended to support regulatory decision making but may not fully capture information of greatest import to patients and prescribers. For patient stakeholders, the most important outcomes include how a person "feels, functions and survives" [1]. These outcomes are often designated as key secondary endpoints.

Clinicians who use the results of clinical trials to inform patient care have a stake in understanding how PROMs are developed and how their psychometric properties are assessed. Key properties include reliability, validity, and sensitivity to change (as defined below). Healthcare professionals use information from package inserts based on PROMs from clinical trials to evaluate treatment options. Many practitioners incorporate PROMs into their clinical practice to improve their understanding of how migraine effects their patients and how treatment addresses those effects. PROMs can be used to track disease symptomology, burden and treatment benefits, facilitate documentation of clinical trajectories, flag concerns, set goals and facilitate patient-professional conversation.

## 4.2 Patient Report Outcomes and Patient Reported Outcome Measures

### 4.2.1 Definitions

A PRO is a report directly from a patient about their health, their symptoms, their functional status, or health related quality of life (HRQoL). PROs may also include a person's subjective assessment of observable aspects of functioning, behaviors or activities. A PROM is a measure (often called a questionnaire, an assessment tool, a scale, or an instrument) used to assess PROs. A PROM can be administered in multiple formats including clinical interviews (in-person, web-platform or telephonic) or self-administered formats (e.g., paper or electronic). If interviews are used, questions should be read exactly as written and participant responses should be precisely recorded.

Guidelines for clinical trials of acute and preventive migraine treatments recommend the inclusion of PROMs as primary clinical trial endpoints [2, 3]. The primary outcomes in migraine trials for both acute treatments (2-h pain freedom and 2-h freedom from the patient-designated most bothersome symptom) and preventive treatments (change in monthly migraine days or 50% responder rates) are PROMs. Although technically accurate, the term PROM is usually not applied to these primary outcomes and is reserved instead for measures that include multiple questions that are combined to assess particular domains of function, such as HRQOL, disability, interference with daily activities, physical and cognitive function, interictal burden, and other aspects of migraine experience.

### 4.2.2  Patient Reported Outcome Measures (PROMs) Used in Migraine Clinical Trials

Some PROMs were created for use in clinical trials, while others were created for clinical practice and later incorporated into trials. The majority of PROMs commonly used in migraine clinical care were not developed using the FDA recommended process, especially the steps including patient involvement in the development process. Haywood et al. conducted a systematic review of 10,903 abstracts of migraine trials and found 46 abstracts that provided evidence for 20 PROMs. Eleven PROMS were specific to the health-related impact of migraine ($n = 5$) or focused on headache ($n = 6$) [4]. The authors reported that the evidence for measurement validity and score interpretation was strongest for the Migraine-Specific Quality of Life Questionnaire (MSQ v2.1), the Headache Impact Test- 6 item (HIT-6), and the Patient Perception of Migraine Questionnaire (PPMQ-R) [5–7]. They also reported that the evidence of reliability was limited, but acceptable for the HIT-6 [8–10].

As part of the Migraine Clinical Outcome Assessment System (MiCOAS), a project funded by the FDA to develop a publicly available set of migraine outcomes and endpoints grounded in patient input, we conducted comprehensive systematic reviews of the migraine literature through October, 2019 to understand what outcomes had been used in acute and preventive migraine clinical trials [11, 12]. Among the 451 blinded, randomized acute treatment trial manuscripts that were published in 1988 or thereafter (following the introduction of the International Classification of Headache Disorders (ICHD) migraine diagnostic classification), the majority reported $\geq 1$ pain-related outcome (430/451, 95.3%) [11, 13]. These were single question PROs. The most common pain PROs were pain relief (310/430, 72.1%), pain freedom (279/430, 64.9%), and headache recurrence (202/43,051, 47.0%). Rescue medication use was also reported in 64.9% of manuscripts (278/430, 64.9%). One or more associated symptoms including nausea, photophobia, and phonophobia were reported in two thirds of manuscripts (299/451, 66.3%). Most bothersome symptoms were only reported in 3.5% (16/451) of manuscripts and it was in the most recent manuscripts as it is a relatively new addition to regulatory guidance. Forty one percent of manuscripts reported on change in disability or impairment associated with an attack (186/451). About a third of the manuscripts (159/451, 35.3%) included PRO instruments. Of the 28 publications that examined $\geq 1$ migraine/headache-related PRO instrument, 60.7% (17/28) included the 24-h

Migraine Specific Quality of Life questionnaire (24-h-MSQoL) and 17.9% (5/28) included the Patient Perception of Migraine Questionnaire- revised scale (PPMQ-R) [6, 14]. The most commonly used non-migraine/headache-specific PRO instrument/ items which were reported in 150 acute migraine trials were related to treatment satisfaction (41/150, 27.3%), treatment efficacy (57/150, 38.0%), and treatment preference (43/150, 28.7%).

Among the 268 blinded, randomized migraine treatment prevention trial manuscripts published in 1988 or later, more than two thirds examined ≥1 migraine-specific single item PRO (184/268, 68.7%), which included number of days with migraine, attacks, total hours, an index (generally combinations of attack duration and pain intensity/severity), headache pain intensity or severity, and attack duration [12]. More than one third (106/268, 39,6%) examined ≥1 headache-specific outcomes which are the same variables as the migraine-specific single item PROs but using the term "headache" instead of "migraine". Half of the manuscripts (136/268, 50.7%) reported results for ≥1 acute/rescue medication use outcomes. Forty percent (108/268, 40.3%) of manuscripts reported on ≥1 migraine/headache-related PRO instrument or measure. Among those, the Migraine Disability Assessment Scale (MIDAS) was the most commonly included PROM (53/108, 49.1%), followed by the Migraine Specific Quality of Life version 2.1 (MSQ v2.1) instrument (34/108, 31.5%) and the Headache Impact Test- 6 item (HIT-6) (33/108, 30.6%) [5, 7, 15, 16]. Less than a quarter (59/268, 22%) of the sample of manuscripts included ≥1 non-migraine/headache-specific PRO items or measures. These included some version of a Patient Global Impression of Change question (PGIC; 15/59, 25.4%), the Short Form-36 Health Survey (SF-36; 14/59, 23.7%) and the Beck Depression Inventory and Beck Depression Inventory II (BDI and BDI-II; 10/59, 16.9%) [17–19].

### 4.2.3  PROMS That Meet Standards for Use in Clinical Trials and Labeling

A small number of PROMs have been judged to fit for purpose by the FDA, the EMA or both and are included in labels of treatments. At the time of this writing, only three migraine-related PROMs have been deemed "Fit for Purpose" by the FDA and are included in labeling for migraine preventive medications. One is the "Role Function-Restrictive" domain subscale of the MSQ version 2.1, which is included in the label for galcanezumab and atogepant [5, 20–24]. The Migraine Physical Function Impact Diary (MPFID) domains of "Impact on Everyday Activities" and "Physical Impairment," are included in the erenumab label in the US [25]. And the Activity Impairment in Migraine Diary (AIM-D) is included in the atogepant label [23, 26]. The EMA has included additional PROMs in migraine treatment labeling [27]. The HIT-6 and the Migraine Disability Assessment Scale (MIDAS) are included in the erenumab EMA label, and the Role Function-Restrictive domain of the MSQ version 2.1 and the Migraine Disability Assessment Scale (MIDAS) are included in EMA galcanezumab labeling [28, 29].

## *4.2.4  How to Develop, Validate and Evaluate PROMs*

### 4.2.4.1  Regulatory Guidance on the Development and Necessary Qualities of PROMs

In 2009, the FDA issued "Guidance for Industry Patient-Reported Outcome Measures: Use in Medical Product Development to Support Labeling Claims" to provide guidance specific to PROMs intended for use in clinical trials [30]. According to this and additional more recent guidance, PROMs included in trials should be patient-centered (reflecting what matters to patients) and include patient input in their development [31]. They must have demonstrated reliability, validity, and sensitivity to change. Reliability refers to consistency of measurement either for the various items of a PROM or across measurement occasions [32, 33]. One form of reliability is internal consistency reliability. It refers to the correlation among the items in a scale. Another form is test-retest reliability, which reflects the level of agreement between closely spaced administrations of a measure. Validity reflects the extent to which a PROM captures what it is intended to measure [34]. Validity is assessed by examining agreement of a novel measure with measures of the same construct (external validity), by comparing performance in groups expected to differ in scores (known group validity) and by its ability to predict relevant outcomes (predictive validity). Sensitivity to change is the ability of the measure to detect changes such as an improvement or deterioration in the clinical condition of the patient.

The scores provided by PROMs must be interpretable and amenable to consistent application [35]. Interpretability is facilitated if the minimally clinically important difference (MCID) is defined. The MCID is "the smallest difference in score in the domain of interest which patients perceive as beneficial and which would mandate, in the absence of troublesome side effects and excessive cost, a change in the patient's management" [36]. A glossary of relevant terminology is provided here: https://www.fda.gov/drugs/development-approval-process-drugs/patient-focused-drug-development-glossary.

In addition, the FDA is developing a series of four methodologically based, patient-focused drug development (PFDD) guidance documents. These documents describe, in a stepwise manner, how stakeholders (patients, researchers, medical product developers, and others) can collect and submit patient experience data and other relevant information from patients and caregivers to be used for regulatory decision-making. At the time of this writing, two of the documents are published and the other two are in development with opportunities for public review and input. (see Table 4.1) [37]. The EMA has a guidance document with many similarities and some important differences from FDA guidance [27]. The EMA also issued a Regulatory Guidance for the Use of Health Related Quality of Life (HRQL) Measures in the Evaluation of Medicinal Products [38]. They defined HRQL as a broad outcome concept that includes, "the patient's subjective perception of the impact of his disease and its treatment(s) on his daily life, physical, psychological and social functioning and well-being" in the context of evaluating treatment benefit.

**Table 4.1** Guidance documents that describe how stakeholders can collect and submit patient experience data and other relevant information from patients and caregivers to be used in medical product development and regulatory decision-making [37]

| Guidance Number and Name | Status |
|---|---|
| Guidance 1: Collecting Comprehensive and Representative Input [52] | Finalized and published. |
| Guidance 2: Methods to Identify What Is Important to Patients Guidance for Industry, Food and Drug Administration Staff, and Other Stakeholders [53] | Finalized and published. |
| Guidance 3: Selecting, Developing, or Modifying Fit-for Purpose Clinical Outcome Assessments (Draft) [54] | A draft document available on the FDA website at the time of this writing. |
| Guidance 4: Incorporating Clinical Outcome Assessments into Endpoints for Regulatory Decision Making (Public Workshop) [55] | A discussion document is available on the FDA website and a public workshop is scheduled at the time of this writing. |

### 4.2.4.2 Phases of PROM Development and Validation

Generally, the PROM development process can be divided into five major phases: the Exploratory Phase, the Qualitative Phase, the Quantitative Observational Phase, the Randomized Trial Validation Phase, and the Implementation Phase. In the Exploratory Phase, PROM developers define a broad area of interest for measurement (e.g., pain, social function, physical function) and conduct a systematic literature review of prior studies on the topic. In the Qualitative Phase, developers gather input from people with the health condition and other stakeholders (e.g., clinicians, family members) to determine the most important aspects of health or function to measure (often called "domains") and the optimal approaches to measurement (e.g., how many questions to ask, what recall interval to use, what response options to offer). The Qualitative Phase is informed by the literature review and stake holder interviews. Once these determinations are made, measure developers create a draft PROM that includes candidate questions (often called "items") and response options to assess the targeted domains. The draft PROM is then tested in people who have the health condition in a process called cognitive debriefing. The goals are to determine whether people with the condition understand the questions, use the response options as intended, consider the PROM to be comprehensive and relevant to their experiences, and do not find the PROM redundant or unduly burdensome. In the Qualitative Phase, focus groups or individual interviews by experts in qualitative research are essential. In the Qualitative Phase a broad range of concepts is explored until "saturation" is reached. Saturation indicates that after a certain number of interviews no new questions, concepts or domains emerge from the qualitative interview. At the end of the qualitative phase, a set of candidate questions is prepared designed to query the domains of greatest interest. The draft PROM is often overinclusive, containing more questions than needed to produce an accurate measure of the target outcome with the goal of engaging in item reduction by selecting the best questions and eliminating the suboptimal questions. Once a draft PROM is developed it is often assessed in another round of Qualitative interviews before moving on to a Quantitative Observational Study.

The Quantitative Observational Phase consists of a study of the PROM in a target population similar to the one to be enrolled in future clinical trials. Baseline and follow-up data are gathered from patients during the observational study and used to assess the performance of the measure as a whole and to understand how individual questions contribute to the final score. Frequency of administration often reflects the intended sampling strategy for a future randomized treatment trial. Scores for the same individual are compared at different time points to assess retest reliability of the PROM. Depending upon the retest interval these analyses may be confined to individuals who show no evidence of change on measures external to the PROM in development. Scores are compared with other already validated measures or in known groups to assess validity. Measures that can be used define treatment success are administered and used to assess external validity and sensitivity to change. At the end of the Quantitative Study test-retest reliability, internal consistency reliable and validity should be assessed. If the Quantitative Study is large and longitudinal, with good external anchor measures MCIDs can be estimated at this stage.

The Randomized Trial Validation Phase is critical for PROMs that will be used in clinical trials of treatment. In this phase, the PROM is used as an outcome measure to assess the benefits of treatment relative to a comparison group (often placebo but sometimes an active comparator). The PROM may undergo refinement on the basis of data gathered in the trial validation. A final MCID can be determined at this phase, usually by using anchor-based methods [39].

Finally, in the Implementation Phase results of the development and validation phase are communicated and ideally the PROM is made available to other interested users. The PROM can be used to communicate important patient-centered aspects of the benefits of treatment.

### 4.2.4.3 How to Interpret PROs in Trials and Clinical Practice

In clinical trials, PROs can be used to determine the success of a treatment by contrasting response of one treatment of interest to a comparator (either placebo or an active comparator). Depending upon the target population and treatment paradigm (e.g., acute versus preventive treatment), analytic strategies are developed to test the desired outcomes. Most often, in a prevention trial, the PROM is measured prior to initiation of active treatment and prior to initiation of placebo treatment. One approach is to compare the magnitude of the treatment for active treatment vs. placebo to determine if statistical separation is achieved. If a MCID has been determined one can determine the proportion of participants achieving the MCID for active treatment and placebo. This approach, often used for 50% responder rates in migraine prevention trials can also be applied to the proportions of people with a clinically meaningful improvement in HRQoL or a clinically meaningful decrement in disability. Details on research guidelines and strategies are reviewed in Chap. 1. A practicing clinician may use information about what PROMs are included in drug labels to match treatments to patient needs and generally guide expectations. There are several PROMs that are useful and available for use in clinical practice that measure a range of constructs. These instruments may be used in clinical practice to track progress (or lack thereof) for patient and provider tracking, electronic health record documentation, and documentation for obtaining treatment coverage among other purposes. Assessment and tracking of constructs can provide a basis for fruitful provider-patient communication and valuable patient self-reflection. Useful constructs for measurement and tracking can be tailor for each individual patient situation but may include disability and impact (as mentioned previously) as well as migraine symptom severity as measured by the migraine symptom severity score (MSSS), allodynia as measured by ASC-12 (ASC-12), interictal burden as measured by migraine interictal burden scale (MIBS-4), depression as measured by 9-item Patient Health Questionnaire (PHQ-9), anxiety as measured by the 7-item generalized anxiety disorder scale (GAD-7), and treatment optimization as measured by migraine treatment optimization questionnaire (mTOQ) [26, 40–46]. These instruments are described in detail in other chapters.

## 4.3   Discussion

PROMs play varied and significant roles in both clinical trials and clinical care of migraine and headache. The FDA and EMA play key roles in determining which PROMs are suitable for inclusion in the regulatory labels for drugs and devices. They highlight the importance of utilizing patient input at each step of development; however, many of the instruments commonly used were developed before the guidance with varying levels of patient input in the development process. Most PROMs for migraine were created for clinical use, though some measures were developed following FDA regulatory guidelines. Clinical trials have primary endpoints which are often specified by regulators but do not necessarily capture what matters most to patients and healthcare professionals such as the commonly used acute endpoint of pain freedom at 2 h post treatment. These endpoints should be psychometrically robust, easy to measure and communicate, but they may or may not reflect what matters most to patients. For example, concepts such as the ability to function and freedom from disability are commonly mentioned by patients in clinical discussions about treatment goals for both acute and preventive treatments. They may also discuss personally bothersome associated symptoms, which are rarely primary endpoints and may be secondary or exploratory endpoints or not included at all.

It is particularly challenging to select the most important measures for migraine trials for several reasons. The primary features of migraine, pain, nausea, photophobia and phonophobia are subjective experiences reported by patients but not amenable to objective verification. In addition, migraine is a symptom complex. The bothersome symptoms are diverse, vary from person to person and within person from attack to attack [47–49]. Migraine is a chronic disorder with episodic manifestations, which also raises the issue of migraine's impact, both during attacks (ictal burden) and between attacks (interictal burden) [50].

Results from the first round of qualitative work from the MiCOAS project found that one area of import, not well captured in current PROMs and brought to light in our qualitative work is the cognitive domain [51]. Most PROMs have no questions or few questions on the cognitive effects of migraine. There is another gap is in the area of ictal versus interictal dysfunction. Most measures focus only on ictal dysfunction, as exemplified by MIDAS, or examine total burden pooling across headache days and headache free days, as exemplified by MPFID, AIM-D and HIT-6.

Clinicians care about what matters to their patients and want to align therapeutic outcomes with patient goals and values. Utilizing PROM data from existing instruments in therapeutic decision making can help healthcare professionals and patients make the best choice for each patient. What is needed in clinical practice is more nuanced based on a broader range of human experience. Multidimensional PROMs that capture a broader range of patient concerns and therapeutic effects that are selected to reflect both patient values and aspects that are essential to clinical decision making are necessary. Future PROM development should attempt to address these gaps for clinical trial use and clinical practice.

In conclusion, PROMs play valuable roles in clinical trials and research. They are necessary for regulatory bodies to interpret the results of clinical trials, especially in a disease such as migraine where there are no objective indicators. There are a small number of PROMs included in product labels, due in part to the requirements that these regulatory bodies place on PROMs to determine that they are "fit for use". There is an extensive process by which a PROM should be developed and tested. There is a need to develop PROMs to address areas of migraine-impact that are commonly reported by patients, but for which there are currently no approved PROMs. Clinical trial results and labeling inclusion of PROMs can be useful to clinicians to match patient needs to particular treatments and set expectations. Clinically, PROMs can play a useful role in treatment assessment, tracking, documentation, and facilitating provider-patient conversation and goal setting.

**Acknowledgements** We would like to thank our colleagues on the MiCOAS project for their thoughtful insights and contributions including RJ Wirth, PhD, Carrie Houts, PhD, Jim McGinley, PhD, Tracy Nishida, PhD, Rikki Mangrum, MLS, and Calvin Hall, PhD.

# References

1. US Department of Health and Human Services F. Center for Drug Evaluation and Research (CDER) and Center for Biologics Evaluation and Research (CBER) Multiple endpoints for clinical trials: guidance for industry. 2022. https://www.fda.gov/media/162416/download
2. Tassorelli C, Diener HC, Dodick DW, et al. Guidelines of the international headache society for controlled trials of preventive treatment of chronic migraine in adults. Cephalalgia. 2018;38:815–32.

 3. Diener HC, Tassorelli C, Dodick DW, et al. Guidelines of the International Headache Society for controlled trials of acute treatment of migraine attacks in adults: fourth edition. Cephalalgia. 2019;38:687–710.
 4. Haywood KL, Mars TS, Potter R, Patel S, Matharu M, Underwood M. Assessing the impact of headaches and the outcomes of treatment: a systematic review of patient-reported outcome measures (PROMs). Cephalalgia. 2018;38:1374–86.
 5. Martin BC, Pathak DS, Sharfman MI, et al. Validity and reliability of the migraine-specific quality of life questionnaire (MSQ version 2.1). Headache. 2000;40:204–16.
 6. Revicki DA, Kimel M, Beusterien K, et al. Validation of the revised patient perception of migraine questionnaire: measuring satisfaction with acute migraine treatment. Headache. 2006;46(2):240–52.
 7. Kosinski M, Bayliss MS, Bjorner JB, et al. A six-item short-form survey for measuring headache impact: the HIT-6™. Qual Life Res. 2003;12:963–74.
 8. Houts CR, McGinley JS, Wirth RJ, Cady R, Lipton RB. Reliability and validity of the 6-item Headache Impact Test in chronic migraine from the PROMISE-2 study. Qual Life Res. 2021;30(3):931–43. https://doi.org/10.1007/s11136-020-02668-2.
 9. Houts CR, Wirth RJ, McGinley JS, Cady R, Lipton RB. Determining thresholds for meaningful change for the headache impact test (HIT-6) total and item-specific scores in chronic migraine. Headache. 2020;60(9):2003–13. https://doi.org/10.1111/head.13946.
10. Houts CR, Wirth RJ, McGinley JS, Gwaltney C, Kassel E, Snapinn S, Cady R. Content validity of HIT-6 as a measure of headache impact in people with migraine: a narrative review. Headache. 2020;60(1):28–39. https://doi.org/10.1111/head.13701.
11. Houts CR, McGinley JS, Nishida TK, et al. Systematic review of outcomes and endpoints in acute migraine clinical trials. Headache. 2021;61(2):263–75.
12. McGinley JS, Houts CR, Nishida TK, et al. Systematic review of outcomes and endpoints in preventive migraine clinical trials. Headache. 2021;61(2):253–62.
13. Headache Classification Committee of the International Headache Society. Classification and diagnostic criteria for headache disorders, cranial neuralgias and facial pain. Cephalalgia. 1988;8:1–96.
14. Hartmaier SL, Santanello NC, Epstein RS, Silberstein SD. Development of a brief 24-hour migraine-specific quality of life questionnaire. Headache. 1995;35(6):320–9.
15. Stewart WF, Lipton RB, Dowson AJ, Sawyer J. Development and testing of the migraine disability assessment (MIDAS) questionnaire to assess headache-related disability. Neurology. 2001;56:S20–8.
16. Jhingran P, Osterhaus JT, Miller DW, Lee JT, Kirchdoerfer L. Development and validation of the migraine-specific quality of life questionnaire. Headache. 1998;38:295–302.
17. Ware JE Jr, Kosinski M, Bjorner JB, Turner-Bowker DM, Gandek B, Maruish ME. User's manual for the SF-36v2® health survey. 2nd ed. Lincoln, RI: Quality Metric Incorporated; 2000.
18. Beck AT, Ward CH, Mendelson M, Mock J, Erbaugh J. An inventory for measuring depression. Arch Gen Psychiatry. 1961;4:561–71.
19. Beck AT, Steer RA, Brown GK. Manual for the Beck depression inventory-II. San Antonio, TX: Psychological Corporation; 1996.
20. Speck RM, Shalhoub H, Ayer DW, Ford JH, Wyrwich KW, Bush EN. Content validity of the migraine-specific quality of life questionnaire version 2.1 electronic patient-reported outcome. J Patient Rep Outcomes. 2019;3:39.
21. Speck RM, Shalhoub H, Wyrwich KW, et al. Psychometric validation of the role function restrictive domain of the migraine specific quality-of-life questionnaire version 2.1 electronic patient-reported outcome in patients with episodic and chronic migraine. Headache. 2019;59:756–74.
22. Speck RM, Yu R, Ford JH, Ayer DW, Bhandari R, Wyrwich KW. Psychometric validation and meaningful within-patient change of the migraine-specific quality of life questionnaire version 2.1 electronic patient-reported outcome in patients with episodic and chronic migraine. Headache. 2021;61:511–26.

23. https://www.accessdata.fda.gov/drugsatfda_docs/label/2021/215206Orig1s000lbl.pdf
24. https://www.accessdata.fda.gov/drugsatfda_docs/label/2018/761063s000lbl.pdf
25. Kawata AK, Hsieh R, Bender R, et al. Psychometric evaluation of a novel instrument assessing the impact of migraine on physical functioning: the migraine physical function impact diary. Headache. 2017;57(9):1385–98.
26. Lipton RB, Gandhi P, Stokes J, et al. Development and validation of a novel patient-reported outcome measure in people with episodic migraine and chronic migraine: the activity impairment in migraine diary. Headache. 2022;62(1):89–105.
27. DeMuro C, Clark M, Doward L, Evans E, Mordin M, Gnanasakthy A. Assessment of PRO label claims granted by the FDA as compared to the EMA (2006–2010). Value Health. 2013;16(8):1150–5.
28. https://www.ema.europa.eu/en/documents/product-information/aimovig-epar-product-information_en.pdf
29. Emgality, INN-galcanezumab (europa.eu). https://www.ema.europa.eu/en/documents/product-information/emgality-epar-product-information_en.pdf
30. Guidance for industry patient-reported outcome measures: use in medical product development to support labeling claims, Guidance for Industry (fda.gov). Accessed 26 Oct 2022.
31. Roadmap to patient-focused outcome measurement in clinical trials. http://www.fda.gov/downloads/Drugs/DevelopmentApprovalProcess/DrugDevelopmentToolsQualificationProgram/UCM370174.pdf. Accessed 26 Oct 2022.
32. Lipton RB, Stewart WF, Merikangas KR. Reliability in headache diagnosis. Cephalalgia. 1993;13(Suppl 12):29–33.
33. Feldt LS, Brennan RL. Reliability. In: Linn RL, editor. Educational measurement. 3rd ed. Macmillan Publishing; American Council on Education; 1989. p. 105–46.
34. Messick S. Validity. In: Linn RL, editor. Educational measurement. 3rd ed. Macmillan Publishing; American Council on Education; 1989. p. 13–103.
35. Coon CD, Cappelleri JC. Interpreting change in scores on patient-reported outcome instruments. Ther Innov Regul Sci. 2016;50(1):22–9.
36. Jaeschke R, Singer J, Guyatt GH. Measurement of health status: ascertaining the minimal clinically important difference. Control Clin Trials. 1989 Dec;10(4):407–15.
37. https://www.fda.gov/drugs/development-approval-process-drugs/fda-patient-focused-drug-development-guidance-series-enhancing-incorporation-patients-voice-medical
38. Reflection Paper on the regulatory guidance for the use of Health Related Quality of Life (HRQL) measures in the evaluation of medicinal products. http://www.ispor.org/workpaper/emea-hrql-guidance.pdf. Accessed 2 Oct 2022.
39. Anvari F, Lakens D. Using anchor-based methods to determine the smallest effect size of interest. J Exp Soc Psychol. 2021;96:104159.
40. Lipton RB, Bigal ME, Ashina S, et al. Cutaneous allodynia in the migraine population. Ann Neurol. 2008;63(2):148–58.
41. Bigal ME, Ashina S, Burstein R, et al. Prevalence and characteristics of allodynia in headache sufferers: a population study. Neurology. 2008;70(17):1525–33.
42. Serrano D, Buse DB, Reed ML, Runken C, Lipton RB. Development of the Migraine Symptom Severity Score (MSSS): a latent variable model for migraine definition. Headache. 2010;50:S40.
43. Buse DC, Rupnow MF, Lipton RB. Assessing and managing all aspects of migraine: migraine attacks, migraine-related functional impairment, common comorbidities, and quality of life. Mayo Clin Proc. 2009;84(5):422–35.
44. Kroenke K, Spitzer RL, Williams JB. The PHQ-9: validity of a brief depression severity measure. J Gen Intern Med. 2001;16(9):606–13.
45. Spitzer RL, Kroenke K, Williams JBW, Löwe B. A brief measure for assessing generalized anxiety disorder: the GAD-7. Arch Intern Med. 2006;166(10):1092–7.
46. Lipton RB, Kolodner K, Bigal ME, et al. Validity and reliability of the migraine-treatment optimization questionnaire. Cephalalgia. 2009;29(7):751–9.

47. McGinley JS, Houts CR, Wirth RJ, Lipton RB. Measuring headache day severity using multiple features in daily diary designs. Cephalalgia. 2022;42(1):53–62.
48. Lipton RB, Dodick DW, Ailani J, McGill L, Hirman J, Cady R. Patient-identified most bothersome symptom in preventive migraine treatment with eptinezumab: a novel patient-centered outcome. Headache. 2021;61(5):766–76.
49. Munjal S, Singh P, Reed ML, et al. Most bothersome symptom in persons with migraine: results from the migraine in America symptoms and treatment (MAST) study. Headache. 2020;60(2):416–29.
50. Haut SR, Bigal ME, Lipton RB. Chronic disorders with episodic manifestations: focus on epilepsy and migraine. Lancet Neurol. 2006;5(2):148–57.
51. Gerstein MT, Wirth RJ, Uzumcu AA, et al. Patient-reported experiences with migraine-related cognitive symptoms—results of the MiCOAS qualitative study. Headache. 2022. In press.
52. Patient-Focused Drug Development: collecting comprehensive and representative input guidance for industry. Food and Drug Administration Staff, and other stakeholders, FDA; 2020. https://www.fda.gov/media/139088/download. Accessed 26 Oct 2022.
53. https://www.fda.gov/media/131230/download
54. https://www.fda.gov/media/159500/download
55. https://www.fda.gov/media/132505/download or https://www.fda.gov/drugs/development-approval-process-drugs/public-workshop-patient-focused-drug-development-guidance-4-incorporating-clinical-outcome

# Chapter 5
# Measuring Pain Intensity in Headache Trials

Rune Häckert Christensen and Faisal Mohammad Amin

## 5.1 Introduction

Pain is a subjective feeling consisting of several inputs, including nociceptive information, previous experiences as well as the emotional and cognitive state of mind. Several attempts to develop objective measurement tools as for instance MRI scans sequences have not established an fully objective method to measure pain. Nevertheless, measurement of pain is invariable in clinical trials of pain and headache treatment. To this end, self-reported pain scales are used. In headache and migraine clinical trial guidelines, such pain scales are taken in part to assess treatment outcomes and endpoints. In general, the available pain scales have excellent psychometric properties, with high reliability and validity between scales [1, 2]. A common limitation is that they are not extensively validated for headache specifically. The scales can be divided into unimodal scales and multimodal scales. Unimodal scales measure pain intensity, while multimodal scales also measure other pain-related variables such as pain quality or interference with daily activities. The most common pain measurement tool in both mentioned categories will be explained in the following.

R. H. Christensen
Department of Neurology, Danish Headache Center, Copenhagen University
Hospital - Rigshospitalet, Copenhagen, Denmark

F. M. Amin (✉)
Department of Neurology, Danish Headache Center, Copenhagen University
Hospital - Rigshospitalet, Copenhagen, Denmark

Department of Brain and Spinal Cord Injury, Copenhagen University
Hospital - Rigshospitalet, Copenhagen, Denmark
e-mail: faisal@dadlnet.dk


P. Yalınay Dikmen, A. Özge (eds.), *Clinical Scales for Headache Disorders*,
Headache, https://doi.org/10.1007/978-3-031-25938-8_5

## 5.2   Unimodal Pain Intensity Scales

The unimodal pain scales are most common in headache research and include the four—and six-point Verbal Rating Scales (VRS), the Numerical Rating Scale (NRS), the Visual Analogue Scale (VAS), and the Faces Pain Scale-Revised (FPS-R).

### 5.2.1   The Four-Point Verbal Rating Scale

The four-point Visual Rating Scale (VRS) is commonly used to grade headache intensity in clinical trials and practice. Pain is rated as none (0 points), mild (1 point), moderate (2 points), or severe (3 points) [3]. Mild pain does not interfere with usual activities, moderate pain inhibits but does not prevent usual activities, while severe pain prohibits all activities, as defined in the International Classification of Headache Disorders, third edition (ICHD-3) [4]. The four-point VRS has high reliability, though this has not been examined for headache [5]. It captures pain intensity in sufficient detail to evaluate all intensity-related primary and secondary outcomes recommended in the IHS guidelines. In clinical trials of acute headache treatment, the four-point VRS is used to grade headache intensity at pre-specified intervals after treatment intake (e.g. 1, 2, or 4 h), while in in trials of preventive treatment, participants record pain intensity daily. The scale is recommended in guidelines of the International Headache Society (IHS) for trials on acute and preventive treatment of both migraine and tension-type headache [6–9].

### 5.2.2   The Six-Point Verbal Rating Scale

A six-point VRS has less commonly been used to grade headache intensity in clinical trials. In the six-point VRS, patients rate pain intensity as none (0 points), mild (1 point), moderate (2 points), severe (3 points), very severe (4 points), or most severe (5 points). These scores are less clearly defined than those of the four-point VRS, which refer to the ICHD-3. The scale has high reliability for acute pain but has not been tested specifically for headache [10]. However, one study found that compared to the four-point VRS, the six-point VRS may have superior correlation with more sensitive pain scales such as the VAS [11]. The six-point is not currently recommended by IHS guidelines for use in clinical trials.

### 5.2.3  The Numerical Rating Scale

In some instances, the VRS is not sensitive enough to detect minor differences in pain intensity. An alternative is the Numerical Rating Scale (NRS), an 11-point scale used to measure pain intensity. Patients rate their pain on a scale from 0 to 10, where 0 represents "no pain" and 10 represents "the worst pain possible". The NRS has excellent reliability and is highly correlated with the four-point VRS, while being more sensitive to differences in pain intensity [2, 5, 12]. The superior sensitivity of the NRS has been validated in migraine patients, where the NRS was 55% more sensitive for clinically important differences in pain intensity than the four-point VRS [13]. The increased sensitivity makes the NRS useful to detect pain intensity changes across repeated measures e.g. in response to treatment or provoking substances, and to correlate pain intensity with other clinical variables. The scale is sometimes converted into the four-point VRS, where 1–3 points on the NRS are graded as mild pain, 4–6 points as moderate, and 7–10 points as severe. However, this approach has not been validated for headache. A possible statistical advantage to using the NRS compared to the four-point VRS is that it provides data which may be analyzed with more powerful, parametric tests, at least when normally distributed [14, 15]. However, it has been debated for decades whether this is statistically valid, since the pain scales consists of ordinal data, which should as a rule only be analyzed with non-parametric tests. The NRS is listed as an alternative to the four-point VRS in the IHS guidelines for trials on acute treatment of migraine [8].

### 5.2.4  The Visual Analogue Scale

The Visual Analogue Scale (VAS) is a continuous scale which scores pain intensity using a measuring instrument [16]. The patients mark the pain intensity on a straight, usually 100-mm line, whose extremes are marked with the anchors "no pain" and "pain as bad as it could be". The distance from mark to the "no pain" anchor is then measured to provide a score between 0 and 100. The reliability of the VAS for acute pain in general is high, but reliability has not been tested for headache specifically [17]. The VAS constitutes the most sensitive tool for detecting differences in pain intensity amongst those presented here. It is available for parametric tests, but it is tedious to apply in practice, since investigators must measure the head pain intensity [5]. Digital versions which automatically measure the distance may help resolve this. Once measured, the intensity can be graded arbitrarily as mild (0–30 mm), moderate (31–69 mm), or severe (70–100 mm) [18]. However, the cut-off values of this grading and the head pain intensity grades defined in the ICHD-3 have not been validated and pose a challenge to interpretation of the VAS in headache research. The correlation between VAS and NRS is high in general but has not been investigated for headache patients specifically [19]. The scale is recommended as an alternative to the four-point VRS in the IHS guidelines for trials of acute treatment of migraine and tension-type-headache [8, 9].

### 5.2.4.1 The Faces Pain Scale-Revised

The Faces Pain Scale-Revised (FPS-R) is an 11-item point scale which rates pain intensity between 0 and 10 points [20]. On the scale, 0 points designate "no pain" and 10 points designate the "very much pain". The scale is anchored with six faces in increasing states of distress. The scale has the advantage of being usable by children from the age of 3 years, and the scale has high reliability across multiple pain states in children [20, 21]. It has an excellent correlation with the VAS scale in adults and children, though this correlation has not been examined specifically in headache [20]. The Faces Scale or equivalents are recommended as an alternative to the four-point VRS in the IHS guidelines for trials on preventive treatment of migraine in children and adolescents [22].

## 5.3 Multimodal Pain Intensity Scales

Pain intensity scales are implemented in several self-administered questionnaires that evaluate multidimensional aspects of pain. These questionnaires are less widely used in headache research, and their use is not emphasized by the current guidelines. They may represent possible future research tools in headache sciences. The multimodal scales include the McGill Pain Questionnaire and the Brief Pain Inventory (BPI).

### 5.3.1 The McGill Pain Questionnaire

The McGill Pain Questionnaire developed by Ronald Melzack assesses pain intensity and quality [23]. It consists of 78-word descriptors categorized into 20 subscales. These address four major domains of pain: sensory, affective, evaluative, and miscellaneous. Furthermore, the questionnaire contains a six-point NRS. Scores are summarized from 0 to 78 points to reach a total score. The questionnaire is available in 26 languages, with minor reliability differences based on language. Within headache research, the questionnaire has occasionally been used to distinguish headache disorders, including tension-type headache, episodic—and chronic migraine based on pain intensity and quality [24–26].

### *5.3.2   Brief Pain Inventory*

The Brief Pain Inventory is a self-administered questionnaire which assesses pain intensity and interference. A 9—and 17-item version is available [27]. The questionnaire follows a two-factor structure, rating pain intensity and pain interference. Pain intensity is investigated using the NRS for four items: the worst pain, the least pain, the average pain, and the current pain. Pain interference is evaluated on 11-point numerical ratings scales of interference. Interference is rated from 0 to 10, where 0 represent "does not interfere" and 10 indicates "completely interferes". Pain interference is rated for seven items related to daily activities: general activities, mood, normal work, walking abilities, relations with other people, sleep, and enjoyment of life. The inventory's use in headache research has this far been limited.

## 5.4   Pain Scales in Clinical Trials and Practice

The pain intensity scales are essential to evaluate outcomes in clinical trials of headache. Pain freedom at 2 h after treatment intake is the recommended primary outcome for acute treatment of migraine and tension-type headache, and relies on changes in pain intensity [8, 9]. Secondary outcomes such as headache intensity and headache relief 2 h after treatment intake are likewise fully dependent on reliable assessment of pain intensity. In trials of preventive treatment of episodic and chronic migraine, change in monthly migraine days and moderate to severe headache days constitute co-primary endpoints that are also contingent on headache intensity scoring [6, 7]. Furthermore, the headache intensity at intake of treatment is likewise of importance. In most trials, patients are asked to treat their migraine headache once it reaches at least moderate intensity, while some trials focus on early treatment while pain is mild.

In clinical practice, pain scales are likewise crucial. The four-point VRS is the pain scale most frequently employed. Recording headache pain intensity and associated symptoms in a headache diary is a widely used and recommended approach to aid headache diagnosis. Furthermore, headache calendars recording intensity of attacks before and after initiation of preventive treatment can be used to monitor therapeutic response [28].

## 5.5   Conclusion

Pain is a subjective feeling but can be assessed based on validated scales. These scales are used to monitor treatment in the clinic as well as in research trials. Clinical trials of headache treatment response are impossible to carry out without assessment of pain intensity. The most used scales are either unimodal or multimodal.

Unimodal only assess pain intensity, whereas multimodal scales also include other outcome measures. The four-point and six-points VRS, the VAS, and NRS are examples of unimodal scales, while the *The McGill Pain Questionnaire* and *Brief Pain Inventory* are among the most used multimodal scales used in headache research.

**Conflicts of Interest** R.H.C. reports no conflicts of interests. F.M.A. has received honoria or personal fees from Pfizer, Teva, Novartis, Lundbeck and Eli Lilly for lecturing or participating in advisory boards; is principal investigator for phase IV trials sponsored by Novartis and by Teva; serves as president of Danish Headache Society and board member of the European Headache Federation; serves as associate editor for Acta Neurol Scand, Front Neurol, Front Res Pain, and Headache Medicine; serves as junior associate editor for Cephalalgia and Cephalalgia Reports; member of the editorial board of J Headache Pain.

# References


1. Jensen MP, Karoly P, Braver S. The measurement of clinical pain intensity: a comparison of six methods. Pain. 1986;27:117–26. https://doi.org/10.1016/0304-3959(86)90228-9.
2. Ferreira-Valente MA, Pais-Ribeiro JL, Jensen MP. Validity of four pain intensity rating scales. Pain. 2011;152:2399–404. https://doi.org/10.1016/J.PAIN.2011.07.005.
3. Handbook of pain assessment. 3rd ed. https://www.guilford.com/books/Handbook-of-Pain-Assessment/Turk-Melzack/9781606239766. Accessed 21 Oct 2022
4. Headache Classification Committee of the International Headache Society (IHS). The international classification of headache disorders, 3rd edition. Cephalalgia. 2018;38:1–211. https://doi.org/10.1177/0333102417738202.
5. Alghadir AH, Anwer S, Iqbal A, Iqbal ZA. Test-retest reliability, validity, and minimum detectable change of visual analog, numerical rating, and verbal rating scales for measurement of osteoarthritic knee pain. J Pain Res. 2018;11:851–6. https://doi.org/10.2147/JPR.S158847.
6. Diener HC, Tassorelli C, Dodick DW, et al. Guidelines of the International Headache Society for controlled trials of preventive treatment of migraine attacks in episodic migraine in adults. Cephalalgia. 2020;40:1026–44. https://doi.org/10.1177/0333102420941839.
7. Tassorelli C, Diener HC, Dodick DW, et al. Guidelines of the International Headache Society for controlled trials of preventive treatment of chronic migraine in adults. Cephalalgia. 2018;38:815–32. https://doi.org/10.1177/0333102418758283.
8. Diener H-C, Tassorelli C, Dodick DW, et al. Guidelines of the International Headache Society for controlled trials of acute treatment of migraine attacks in adults: Fourth edition. Cephalalgia. 2020;41(11–12):1135–51. https://doi.org/10.1177/0333102419828967.
9. Bendtsen L, Bigal ME, Cerbo R, et al. Guidelines for controlled trials of drugs in tension-type headache: second edition. Cephalalgia. 2009;30:1–16. https://doi.org/10.1111/J.1468-2982.2009.01948.X.
10. Jensen MP, Miller L, Fisher LD. Assessment of pain during medical procedures: a comparison of three scales. Clin J Pain. 1998;14:343–9. https://doi.org/10.1097/00002508-199812000-00012.
11. Aicher B, Peil H, Peil B, Diener HC. Pain measurement: Visual Analogue Scale (VAS) and Verbal Rating Scale (VRS) in clinical trials with OTC analgesics in headache. Cephalalgia. 2012;32:185–97. https://doi.org/10.1177/0333102411430856.
12. Ekblom A, Hansson P. Pain intensity measurements in patients with acute pain receiving afferent stimulation. J Neurol Neurosurg Psychiatry. 1988;51:481–6. https://doi.org/10.1136/JNNP.51.4.481.

13. Kwong WJ, Pathak DS. Validation of the eleven-point pain scale in the measurement of migraine headache pain. Cephalalgia. 2007;27:336–42. https://doi.org/10.1111/J.1468-2982 .2007.01283.X.
14. Nair AS, Diwan S. Pain scores and statistical analysis—the conundrum. Ain-Shams J Anesthesiol. 2020;121(12):1–2. https://doi.org/10.1186/S42077-020-00085-8.
15. McCormack HM, Horne DJ, Sheather S. Clinical applications of visual analogue scales: a critical review. Psychol Med. 1988;18:1007–19. https://doi.org/10.1017/S0033291700009934.
16. Huskisson EC. Measurement of pain. Lancet. 1974;2:1127–31. https://doi.org/10.1016/ S0140-6736(74)90884-8.
17. Bijur PE, Silver W, Gallagher EJ. Reliability of the visual analog scale for measurement of acute pain. Acad Emerg Med. 2001;8:1153–7. https://doi.org/10.1111/J.1553-2712.2001. TB01132.X.
18. Kelly AM. The minimum clinically significant difference in visual analogue scale pain score does not differ with severity of pain. Emerg Med J. 2001;18:205–7. https://doi.org/10.1136/ EMJ.18.3.205.
19. Thong ISK, Jensen MP, Miró J, Tan G. The validity of pain intensity measures: what do the NRS, VAS, VRS, and FPS-R measure? Scand J Pain. 2018;18:99–107. https://doi.org/10.1515/ SJPAIN-2018-0012.
20. Hicks CL, Von Baeyer CL, Spafford PA, et al. The Faces Pain Scale-Revised: toward a common metric in pediatric pain measurement. Pain. 2001;93:173–83. https://doi.org/10.1016/ S0304-3959(01)00314-1.
21. Tomlinson D, Von Baeyer CL, Stinson JN, Sung L. A systematic review of faces scales for the self-report of pain intensity in children. Pediatrics. 2010;126:e1168–98. https://doi. org/10.1542/PEDS.2010-1609.
22. Abu-Arafeh I, Hershey AD, Diener HC, Tassorelli C. Guidelines of the International Headache Society for controlled trials of preventive treatment of migraine in children and adolescents: first edition. Cephalalgia. 2019;39:803–16. https://doi.org/10.1177/0333102419842188.
23. Melzack R. The McGill Pain Questionnaire: major properties and scoring methods. Pain. 1975;1:277–99. https://doi.org/10.1016/0304-3959(75)90044-5.
24. Allen RA, Weinmann RL. The mcGill-Melzack Pain Questionnaire in the diagnosis of headache. Headache. 1982;22:20–9. https://doi.org/10.1111/J.1526-4610.1982.HED2201020.X.
25. Mongini F, Deregibus A, Raviola F, Mongini T. Confirmation of the distinction between chronic migraine and chronic tension-type headache by the McGill Pain Questionnaire. Headache. 2003;43:867–77. https://doi.org/10.1046/J.1526-4610.2003.03165.X.
26. Hunter M, Philips C. The experience of headache pain—an assessment of the qualities of tension headache pain. Pain. 1981;10:209–19. https://doi.org/10.1016/0304-3959(81)90196-2.
27. Cleeland C, Ryan K. Pain assessment: global use of the Brief Pain Inventory. Ann Acad Med Singap. 1994;23(2):129–38.
28. Eigenbrodt AK, Ashina H, Khan S, et al. Diagnosis and management of migraine in ten steps. Nat Rev Neurol. 2021;178(17):501–14. https://doi.org/10.1038/s41582-021-00509-5.

# Chapter 6
# Clinical Instruments for Diagnosing and Screening of Headache and Migraine

Thien Phu Do and Messoud Ashina

## Abbreviations

| | |
|---|---|
| BHS | Brief Headache Screen |
| CHAT | Computerized Headache Assessment Tool |
| ICHD | International Classification of Headache Disorders |
| ID-CM | Identify Chronic Migraine |
| MS-Q | Migraine Screen Questionnaire |

## 6.1  Introduction

Primary headache disorders are the most common reasons for a neurological consultation. One of the most prevalent headache disorders is migraine and it affects more than 1 billion individuals in the world [1]. As there are no validated biomarkers for primary headache disorders, diagnosis for these diseases rely on the medical history with possible assistance of a range of screening tools. Physical examination is most often normal and conducted for confirmation, whereas further investigations (e.g., neuroimaging) are indicated if a secondary aetiology is suspected and must be confirmed or rejected [2–5]. A rational clinical approach to headache diagnosis is to first exclude secondary aetiology and then afterwards provide a primary headache disorder diagnosis if relevant [2]. However, there will be situations where time restraints, e.g., primary care, or specific setups, e.g., epidemiological research,

T. P. Do · M. Ashina (✉)
Danish Headache Center, Department of Neurology, Rigshospitalet Glostrup, Faculty of
Health and Medical Sciences, University of Copenhagen, Copenhagen, Denmark
e-mail: ashina@dadlnet.dk


P. Yalınay Dikmen, A. Özge (eds.), *Clinical Scales for Headache Disorders*,
Headache, https://doi.org/10.1007/978-3-031-25938-8_6

warrant use of diagnostic screening tools that allow for rapid identification of a specific subpopulation with a relatively high sensitivity and specificity. In this Chapter, we focus on clinical instruments for diagnosing and screening of headache and migraine. We also highlight red flags, green flags, and screening tools for headache.

## 6.2 The International Classification of Headache Disorders

Diagnostic criteria for headache disorders are provided by *The International Classification of Headache Disorders*, third edition (ICHD-3) [6]. *The International Headache Society* developed the ICHD-criteria to harmonize diagnosis of headache disorders across regions; this was of particular interest for researchers as it allowed for consistent and comparative data. For the same reason, the ICHD-3 prioritizes specificity over sensitivity, so additional set of criteria are provided for "probable" diagnoses such as "migraine-like attacks" that can be confirmed during a follow-up. In the ICHD-3, headache disorders are broadly categorized as primary headache disorders—symptoms are due to an inherent pathophysiology—and secondary headache disorders—symptoms are secondary to an external factor, e.g., stroke. The primary headache disorders include migraine, tension-type headache, trigeminal autonomic cephalalgias, and other primary headache disorders. Migraine is classified into three main types: migraine without aura, migraine with aura, and chronic migraine.

### 6.2.1 *Migraine Without Aura*

Migraine without aura is the most common main type and is characterized by recurrent headache episodes of 4–72 h duration [6]. Typical clinical features of an attack include unilateral localization, pulsating quality, moderate or severe pain intensity, and aggravation by routine physical activity [6, 7]. The most common accompanying symptoms consist of photophobia, phonophobia, nausea, and vomiting [7]. For the same reason, the above mentioned features constitute the diagnostic criteria for migraine without aura.

### 6.2.2 *Migraine with Aura*

One-third of individuals with migraine will experience migraine aura, transient focal neurological symptoms that usually precede the headache phase of a migraine attack [6]. The most common presentation is visual symptoms as fortification spectra [8], but other symptoms such as sensory disturbances, e.g., gradually spreading unilateral paraesthesia, is not uncommon [8]. Rarer aura symptoms include motor weakness, retinal symptoms, and brainstem-associated symptoms [9].

### 6.2.3  Chronic Migraine

Chronic migraine is defined as a headache frequency of ≥15 headache days per month with ≥8 of these days fulfilling the criteria for migraine for >3 months [6]. Of note, diagnosis of episodic and chronic migraine is not a static entity and progression to chronic or reversion back to episodic is not uncommon [10].

## 6.3  Primary or Secondary Etiology: Red and Green Flags in Headache

In most cases, patients will have a primary headache disorder with only a minority of presentations being related to a secondary etiology. This will result in wastage due to unnecessary referrals to further diagnostic workup; only a marginal proportion (<6%) of neuroimaging for headache as the primary complaint in the emergency department reveal pathological findings [11]. However, serious secondary pathology should always be excluded. In this context, several diagnostic aids exist that can facilitate identification and stratification of these individuals. A special interest group of *The International Headache Society* developed lists of red flags (indication of secondary etiology) and green flags (indication of primary etiology) [4, 5].

### 6.3.1  Red Flags (SNNOOP10)

The SNOOP mnemonic (systemic symptoms/signs and disease, neurologic symptoms or signs, onset sudden or onset after the age of 40 years, and change of headache pattern) was promoted as a systematic red flag detection tool, and has since been expanded with additional screening items from national and regional guidelines to create the *SNNOOP10* list [4, 12]. *SNNOOP10* covers 15 red flags in headache, their related secondary etiology, and contextualize usage with brief clinical information (Table 6.1). Presence of red flags may warrant further investigations whereas their absence may indicate that no further diagnostic workup is needed. Nonetheless, large case series of patients with pre-existing and diagnosed secondary headache disorders comprise the basis of many red flags, which only allows for the sensitivity to be known. Subsequently, large-scale prospective studies are needed to clarify specificity and predictivity of these red flags.

**Table 6.1** The SNNOOP10 list of red flags for secondary headache disorders

|  | Sign or symptom | Related secondary etiology | Key points |
|---|---|---|---|
| 1 | Systemic symptoms including fever | Headache attributed to infection or non-vascular intracranial disorders, carcinoid or pheochromocytoma. | Headache with fever is primarily alarming when accompanied by relevant symptoms (e.g., neck stiffness, decreased consciousness, and neurologic deficit). |
| 2 | Neoplasm in history | Neoplasms of the brain; metastasis. | A newly developed headache in a patient with neoplasm is highly suspect for an intracranial metastasis. |
| 3 | Neurological deficit or dysfunction (including decreased consciousness) | Headaches attributed to vascular, non-vascular intracranial disorders. Brain abscess and other infections. | Headache occurs in one-fourth of episodes of acute stroke. The severity of headache is not related to the size of the lesion. |
| 4 | Onset of headache is sudden or abrupt (thunderclap headache) | Subarachnoid hemorrhage and other headaches attributed to cranial or cervical vascular disorders. | Thunderclap headache can be the only initial symptom of subarachnoid hemorrhage. |
| 5 | Older age (after 50 years) | Giant cell arteritis and other headache attributed to cranial or cervical vascular disorders. Neoplasms and other non-vascular intracranial disorders. | Older individuals with headache have a higher frequency of secondary etiology. The incidence of primary headache disorders is also lower in this age group. |
| 6 | Pattern change or recent onset of headache | Neoplasms, headaches attributed to vascular, non-vascular intracranial disorders. | A recent change of pattern or a newly developed headache can be the only signs of a secondary etiology. Diagnosis is often delayed in these cases. |
| 7 | Positional headache | Intracranial hypertension or hypotension. | Positional headache is the trademark of intracranial hypotension, and the most common cause is cerebrospinal fluid leak at the spinal level. |
| 8 | Precipitated by sneezing, coughing or exercise | Posterior fossa lesions, Chiari malformation. | Cough headache is highly predictive of Chiari malformations and posterior fossa lesions. |
| 9 | Papilledema | Neoplasms and other non-vascular intracranial disorders; intracranial hypertension. | A high prevalence of patients with papilledema has a serious underlying pathology. |
| 10 | Progressive headache and atypical presentations | Neoplasms and other non-vascular intracranial disorders. | Progressive headache and atypical headache presentation can be the only signs of serious underlying pathology. |

**Table 6.1**  (continued)

|    | Sign or symptom | Related secondary etiology | Key points |
|----|-----------------|---------------------------|------------|
| 11 | Pregnancy or puerperium | Headaches attributed to cranial or cervical vascular disorders; post-dural puncture headache; hypertension related disorders (e.g., preeclampsia); cerebral venous thrombosis; hypothyroidism; anemia; diabetes. | Headache during pregnancy and puerperium has a higher risk of severe pathology. More than one-third of individuals presenting to acute care with headache during pregnancy will have a secondary etiology. Most common causes are hypertensive disorders followed by pituitary adenoma or stroke. Other risk factors are no prior headache history, occurring during third trimester, seizures, hypertension, and fever. |
| 12 | Painful eye with autonomic features | Pathology in posterior fossa, pituitary region or cavernous sinus. Tolosa-Hunt syndrome. Ophthalmic causes. | Patients with presentations of painful eye with autonomic features should undergo neuroimaging as it can be due to a structural lesion. Even typical presentations of cluster headache (or other trigeminal autonomic cephalalgias) can derive from a structural lesion. |
| 13 | Posttraumatic onset of headache | Acute and chronic posttraumatic headache; subdural hematoma and other headache attributed to vascular disorders. | Headache related to trauma should always be explored. |
| 14 | Pathology of the immune system such as AIDS (acquired immunodeficiency syndrome) or medical immunosuppression | Opportunistic infections. | Risk of severe pathology is dependent on the degree of immunosuppression. |
| 15 | Painkiller overuse or new drug at onset of headache | Medication overuse headache; drug incompatibility. | Medication overuse is the most common cause of secondary headache. Onset of headache due to a new drug can be a sign of incompatibility with the given drug. |

Red flags are information that encourage further investigation of a secondary etiology. See: [2, 4]

### 6.3.2  Green Flags

To date, no validated biomarkers have been discovered for primary headache disorders in humans. As an alternative, the concept of green flags was introduced in 2021 (Table 6.2) [5]. Green flags are information indicative of a primary headache disorder. A priority of red flags is to have a high sensitivity for a secondary etiology, a

**Table 6.2** The proposed list of green flags for headache disorders

| | Sign or symptom | Key points |
|---|---|---|
| 1 | The current headache has already been present during childhood | Viral infections are the most common cause of secondary headache in children. In children with chronic headache, the pain is rarely secondary. A life-threatening headache is very unlikely in adults in whom that headache type has already been present during childhood. |
| 2 | The patient has headache-free days | Most primary headache disorders are paroxysmal. Although recurring secondary headache also occur, they are often caused by trigger factors, such as injury to the head, cerebral ischemia, intracranial hemorrhage, arteritis, arterial dissection, or exposure to a substance, e.g., phosphodiesterase inhibitors or nitric oxide donors. An important exception are intracranial tumors that can also present with recurring headache. |
| 3 | The headache occurs in temporal relationship with the menstrual cycle | The relationship between pain and menstrual cycle has been validated with a headache diary. Migraine attacks associated with fluctuations in the menstrual cycle is common. |
| 4 | Close family members have the same headache phenotype | There is a genetic disposition to migraine, cluster headache, and medication overuse headache. The prevalence of genetic vasculopathies is lower than the beforementioned headache disorders. |
| 5 | Headache occurred or stopped more than 1 week ago | Life-threatening secondary headache generally present within few days. Consequently, the more time passed since the headache, the smaller the probability of a life-threatening cause. However, time passed since onset is unlikely to influence the likelihood of other non-life-threatening secondary causes, e.g., temporomandibular disorder, persistent post-traumatic headache. |

Green flags are information that may suggest that no further investigations for a secondary etiology is needed. See: [2, 5]

high sensitivity results in a low number of missed cases. For green flags, the priority is to have a high specificity as this results in a higher number of identified primary headache disorders without missing cases with a secondary etiology. Like *SNNOOP10*, these green flags still need to be confirmed in prospective studies. Even so, can be utilized in cases where reassurance is needed that a headache is a primary headache disorder in the absence of red flags.

### *6.3.3 Red Flags and Green Flags in Clinical Practice*

Both red flags and green flags are physician-administered tools, i.e., requires interview of the patient by a qualified clinician. As red flags are not pathognomonic for their related disorders, the absence of these does not necessarily exclude a secondary etiology, and green flags can be screened for in addition to red flags and whether diagnostic criteria for a primary headache disorder are met according to the ICHD-3

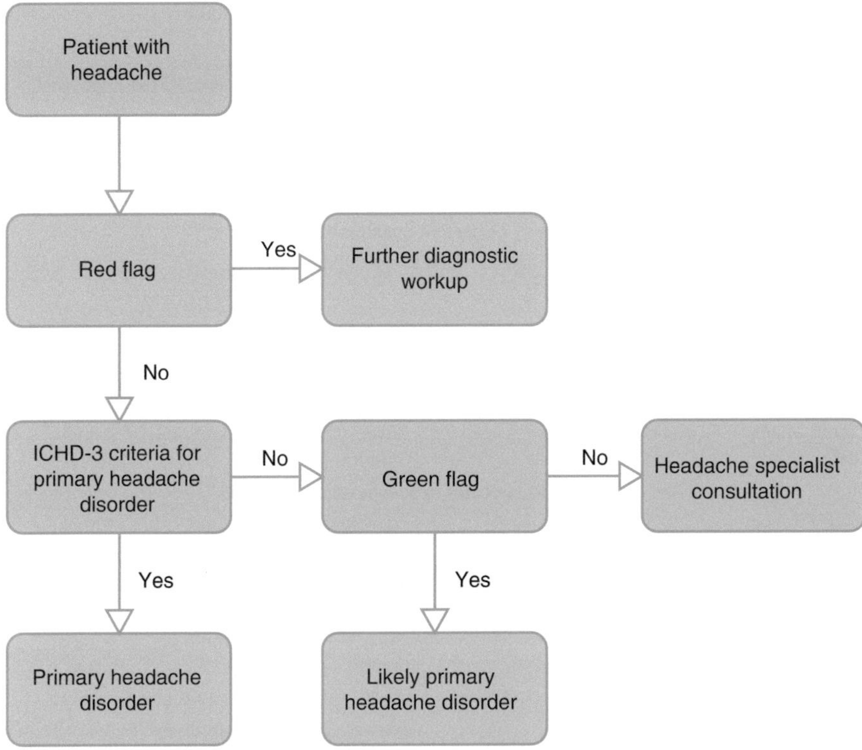


**Fig. 6.1** Systematic approach to diagnosing headache disorders. The SNNOOP10 list can be used to screen patients with headache for red flags. Green flags are information indicative of a primary headache disorder. If both red and green flags are absent without fulfilling ICHD-criteria for a primary headache disorder, consultation with a senior colleague or specialist should be considered. See: [2]

(Fig. 6.1) [6]. If both red and green flags are absent without fulfilling ICHD-criteria for a primary headache disorder, consultation with a senior colleague or specialist should be considered.

## 6.4    Screening Tools for Headache

Several tools exist for rapid and sensitive screening of individuals with headache (Table 6.3). These can be used in settings where time restraints limit deep phenotyping of patients, e.g., the emergency department and general practice. In the context of epidemiological research, these instruments allow for large-scale screening and recruitment of participants. We present a selection of these screening tools.

**Table 6.3** Selection of diagnostic screening tools for headache and migraine

| Screening tool | Format |
| --- | --- |
| Brief Headache Screen (BHS) | Six-item questionnaire; only three of the items are related to diagnosis. |
| Computerized Headache Assessment Tool (CHAT) | Internet-based program with branching logic. |
| ID Migraine Screener | Three-item questionnaire. |
| Identify Chronic Migraine (ID-CM) | 12-item questionnaire. |
| Migraine Screen Questionnaire (MS-Q) | Five-item questionnaire. |

**Table 6.4** Brief headache screen

| 1 | **How often do you get severe headaches (difficult or unable to continue normal function)?** | | | |
| --- | --- | --- | --- | --- |
| Daily or near daily | 3–4 days/week | 2/week–2/month | 1/month or less | Almost never |
| 2 | **How often do you get mild or less severe headaches?** | | | |
| Daily or near daily | 3–4 days/week | 2/week–2/month | 1/month or less | Almost never |
| 3 | **How often do you take pain relievers, or any medication to relieve headache symptoms?** | | | |
| Daily or near daily | 3–4 days/week | 2/week–2/month | 1/month or less | Almost never |
| 4 | How often do you miss some work or leisure time because of headache? | | | |
| Daily or near daily | 3–4 days/week | 2/week–2/month | 1/month or less | Almost never |
| 5 | Are you satisfied with the current medication you use to relieve your headaches? | | | |
| Yes | No | | | |
| 6 | Are you taking daily prescription medicine to prevent headaches? | | | |
| Yes | No | | | |
| | If no, do your headaches trouble you enough to take daily preventive medication? | | | |
| Yes | No | | | |

The Brief Headache Screen consists of a diagnostic segment and a treatment evaluation segment. The diagnostic segment is a three-item questionnaire (**bold**) that interrogates on frequencies of (1) severe (disabling) headache, (2) mild headache, and (3) use of symptomatic medication. See: [13]

## 6.4.1 Brief Headache Screen (BHS)

The Brief Headache Screen is a patient-reported tool developed to screen for migraine and medication overuse and evaluate patient satisfaction with pharmacological treatment (Table 6.4) [13]. It consists of a diagnostic segment and a treatment evaluation segment. The diagnostic segment is a three-item questionnaire that interrogates on frequencies of (1) severe (disabling) headache, (2) mild headache, and (3) use of symptomatic medication. The single criterion of episodic severe (disabling) headache "How often do you experience severe headaches?" had a sensitivity of 0.84 (95% CI, 0.80–0.88) and a specificity of 0.63 (95% CI, 0.49–0.75) for migraine in a pooled cohort of 394 patients from primary care, emergency department, and referral headache clinic [13]. Of note, the sensitivity of the episodic severe (disabling) headache for chronic migraine was lower than for episodic migraine, 0.78 (95% CI, 0.72–0.83) and 0.93 (95% CI, 0.88–0.96) respectively [13].

### 6.4.2  Computerized Headache Assessment Tool (CHAT)

Computerized Headache Assessment Tool is a patient-reported internet-based program that was developed to screen for all major primary headache disorders, distinguish daily from episodic types, and medication overuse [14]. It consists of four sections: an explanatory/disclaimer page, interview section, feedback/summary section, and diagnostic outcome. The questionnaire employs a branching logic, i.e., only relevant questions are presented dependent on prior answers. In an adult urgent care department, the diagnostic tool correctly identified 104/118 (0.88 [95% CI, 0.81–0.93]) cases and correctly identified all patients with episodic migraine, chronic tension-type headache, episodic tension-type headache, and episodic cluster headache [14].

### 6.4.3  ID Migraine Screener

The ID Migraine Screener is a patient-reported three-item screening tool for migraine [15]. The three-item questionnaire interrogates on nausea, photophobia, and disability (Table 6.5). It is positive if $\geq$2 items are fulfilled. In a validation study with a cohort of 563 patients presenting for routine primary care appointments, it had a sensitivity of 0.81 (95% CI, 0.77–0.85) and a specificity of 0.75 (95% CI,

**Table 6.5**  ID Migraine Screener

| During the past 3 months, did you have the following with your headaches? | |
| --- | --- |
| 1 | You felt nauseated or sick to your stomach? |
| Yes | No |
| 2 | Light bothered you (a lot more than when you don't have headaches)? |
| Yes | No |
| 3 | Your headaches limited your ability to work, study, or do what you needed to do? |
| Yes | No |

The three-item ID Migraine Screener interrogates on nausea, photophobia, and disability. It is positive if $\geq$2 items are fulfilled. See: [15]

0.64–0.84). A later systematic review with meta-analysis of 13 studies with 5866 patients had a pooled sensitivity estimate of 0.84 (95% CI, 0.75–0.90) and specificity of 0.76 (95% CI, 0.69–0.83 [16].

### 6.4.4  Identify Chronic Migraine (ID-CM)

The Identify Chronic Migraine questionnaire is a patient-reported screening tool developed to identify individuals with severe headache who have migraine, and amongst those, identify the individuals with chronic migraine [17]. It is a 12-item questionnaire that interrogates on frequency, associated symptoms, medication use, disability, and planning disruption. A validation study demonstrated a sensitivity of 0.81 (95% CI, 0.70–0.88) and a specificity of 0.89 (95% CI, 0.76–0.95) [17]. During development of the 12-item questionnaire, a shorter 6-item variant also demonstrated potential as a good case-finding tool for chronic migraine, but the 12-item variant was favored due to a higher sensitivity and additional data on medication overuse and headache impact [17]. Even so, the six-item variant has demonstrated a high level of specificity, 0.93 (95% CI, 0.81–0.99) and moderate sensitivity, 0.71 (95% CI, 0.58–0.81) in a real-world setting [18].

### 6.4.5  Migraine Screen Questionnaire (MS-Q)

The Migraine Screen Questionnaire is a patient-reported screening tool for migraine [19]. It consists of five items on frequency of headache, duration of headache, nausea, photophobia and phonophobia, and disability (Table 6.6). A validation study

**Table 6.6** Migraine screen questionnaire

| | |
|---|---|
| INSTRUCTIONS: The questions below refer to the headaches or migraine episodes without headache that you may have experienced in your lifetime. Answer each question as indicated. If you are not sure how to answer a given question, please answer what you believe is most correct. | |
| 1 | Do you have frequent or intense headaches? |
| Yes | No |
| 2 | Do your headaches usually last more than 4 h? |
| Yes | No |
| 3 | Do you usually suffer from nausea when you have a headache? |
| Yes | No |
| 4 | Does light or noise bother you when you have a headache? |
| Yes | No |
| 5 | Does headache limit any of your physical or intellectual activities? |
| Yes | No |

See: [19]

**Table 6.7** The Erwin test for cluster headache

| The Erwin test for cluster headache | |
| --- | --- |
| 1 | Is this the worst pain you have ever experienced? |
| Yes | No |
| 2 | Imagine setting a timer. Does the last less than 4 h? |
| Yes | No |
| 3 | During a headache, do one or more of these happen to you?<br>• your eye turns red on only one side<br>• your eye waters on only one side<br>• your nose runs on only one side<br>• your nose gets congested on only one side |
| Yes | No |

A validation study demonstrated a sensitivity is 0.84 (95% CI, 0.73–0.92) and a specificity of 0.89 (95% CI, 0.84–0.94) if all three items are fulfilled. See: [21]

reported that a cut-off point of $\geq$4/5 points provided a sensitivity of 0.93 (95% CI, 0.87–0.99) and specificity of 0.81 (95% CI, 0.72–0.91). Of note, the question on photophobia was the most specific but also least sensitive item, whereas disability had the highest sensitivity [19]. These findings were later reproduced in 9670 patients derived from 410 primary care centres in Spain; here, the sensitivity was 0.82 (95% CI, 0.81–0.84) and specificity 0.97 (95% CI, 0.98–0.99) [20].

### 6.4.6 The Erwin Test for Cluster Headache (ETCH)

The Erwin Test is a patient-reported three-item screening tool for cluster headache [21]. The three-item questionnaire interrogates on the pain intensity, duration, and accompanying autonomic symptoms (Table 6.7). A validation study reported a sensitivity of 0.84 (95% CI, 0.73–0.92) and a specificity of 0.89 (95% CI, 0.84–0.94) [21].

## 6.5 Conclusions

Several diagnostic aids and screening tools exist for headache and migraine, but only a limited number of these have been validated in large populations, other languages, and at different levels of systems of care (e.g., primary care, specialist care, emergency department). The heterogeneity of headache disorders also provides a challenge as more items will be necessary to capture additional diagnoses, which in turn results in a longer survey duration and increased survey attrition. While several of these tools are useful and have already been introduced to clinical practice and research, further development and validation is warranted.

 

# References


1. Ashina M, Buse DC, Ashina H, et al. Migraine: integrated approaches to clinical management and emerging treatments. Lancet. 2021;397:1505–18.
2. Do TP, la Cour Karottki NF, Ashina M. Updates in the diagnostic approach of headache. Curr Pain Headache Rep. 2021;25:80.
3. Eigenbrodt AK, Ashina H, Khan S, et al. Diagnosis and management of migraine in ten steps. Nat Rev Neurol. 2021;17:501–14.
4. Do TP, Remmers A, Schytz HW, et al. Red and orange flags for secondary headaches in clinical practice. Neurology. 2019;92:134–44.
5. Pohl H, Do TP, García-Azorín D, et al. Green flags and headache: a concept study using the Delphi method. Headache. 2021;61:300–9.
6. Anon. Headache classification Committee of the International Headache Society (IHS) the international classification of headache disorders. Cephalalgia. 2018;38:1–211.
7. Rasmussen BK, Jensen R, Schroll M, et al. Epidemiology of headache in a general population – a prevalence study. J Clin Epidemiol. 1991;44:1147–57.
8. Russell MB, Olesen J. A nosographic analysis of the migraine aura in a general population. Brain. 1996;119:355–61.
9. Yamani N, Chalmer MA, Olesen J. Migraine with brainstem aura: defining the core syndrome. Brain. 2019;142:3868–75.
10. Serrano D, Lipton RB, Scher AI, et al. Fluctuations in episodic and chronic migraine status over the course of 1 year: implications for diagnosis, treatment and clinical trial design. J Headache Pain. 2017;18:101.
11. Goldstein J, Camargo C, Pelletier A, et al. Headache in United States emergency departments. Cephalalgia. 2006;26:684–90.
12. Dodick DW. Clinical clues and clinical rules: primary vs secondary headache. Adv Stud Med. 2003;3:87–92.
13. Maizels M, Burchette R. Rapid and sensitive paradigm for screening patients with headache in primary care settings. Headache. 2003;43:441–50.
14. Maizels M, Wolfe WJ. An expert system for headache diagnosis: the Computerized Headache Assessment Tool (CHAT). Headache. 2008;48(1):72–8.
15. Lipton RB, Dodick D, Sadovsky R, et al. A self-administered screener for migraine in primary care. Neurology. 2003;61:375–82.
16. Cousins G, Hijazze S, Van de Laar FA, et al. Diagnostic accuracy of the ID Migraine: a systematic review and meta-analysis. Headache. 2011;51:1140–8.
17. Lipton RB, Serrano D, Buse DC, et al. Improving the detection of chronic migraine: development and validation of identify chronic migraine (ID-CM). Cephalalgia. 2016;36:203–15.
18. Pavlovic JM, Yu JS, Silberstein SD, et al. Evaluation of the 6-item identify chronic migraine screener in a large medical group. Headache. 2021;61:335–42.
19. Láinez MJA, Domínguez M, Rejas J, et al. Development and validation of the Migraine Screen Questionnaire (MS-Q). Headache. 2005;45:1328–38.
20. Láinez MJ, Castillo J, Domínguez M, et al. New uses of the Migraine Screen Questionnaire (MS-Q): validation in the primary care setting and ability to detect hidden migraine. MS-Q in Primary Care. BMC Neurol. 2010;10:39.
21. Parakramaweera R, Evans RW, Schor LI, et al. A brief diagnostic screen for cluster headache: creation and initial validation of the Erwin test for cluster headache. Cephalalgia. 2021;41:1298–309.

# Chapter 7
# Clinical Instruments for Disability, Impact and Burden in Headache and Migraine

Seden Demirci and Derya Uludüz

## 7.1 Introduction

Headaches are one of the most prevailing ailments influencing the population with the global prevalence of 47% of which migraine and tension-type headache (TTH) are the most frequently encountered conditions. Global Burden of Diseases, Injuries and Risk Factors study (GBD) 2016 annunciated nearly 3 billion people affected by TTH or migraine. Approximately 3% of adult population have experience headache on $\geq 15$ days/month [1]. Aforementioned disorders lead to significant disability worldwide, impairing quality of life, damaging productivity, and substantial burdens of financial cost on both the individuls and societies [2]. In GBD study 2019, headache disorders have been estimated to account for 46.6 million years lived with disability (YLDs) globally, which has been 5.4% of all YLDs, with 88.2% of them attributed to migraine [3].

These disorders have ranked as the third motive of disability among the 369 diseases for both genders (following back ache and depressive disorders), and the first reason of disability in adults under the age of 50 [4, 5].

Migraine is a vital health issue in societies in terms of its effects on both the individual and society as a whole. It directly affects more than 1 billion people across the world and constitutes a leading cause of disability [6]. Migraine attacks may disrupt working and academic performance, ability to perform household chores as well as social and pastime activities [7]. Migraine is related to impaired quality of life (QoL) and causes substantial burden not only on patients but also on

S. Demirci
Department of Neurology, School of Medicine, Akdeniz University, Antalya, Turkey

D. Uludüz (✉)
Department of Neurology, Cerrahpaşa School of Medicine, Istanbul University, Istanbul, Turkey



P. Yalınay Dikmen, A. Özge (eds.), *Clinical Scales for Headache Disorders*, Headache, https://doi.org/10.1007/978-3-031-25938-8_7

their families, friends, employers, and co-workers frequently asked for compensating for the absenteeism and reduced effectivity due to headaches and their outcomes. Even once the attack passes, the burden continues to exist, as most patients worry that next attack might be triggered expanding the inability to the headache-free days. Patients with migraine might not admit challenges and responsibilities of the work and might be unwilling to make social and family plans. The major importance of this interictal burden is due to its unpredictable recurrence [1].

As the burden peaks between the ages of 35 and 39, migraine has been considered as the major motive of disability in individuals under the age of 50 worldwide, particularly women. As a result, migraine mainly influence individuals in their productive peak, on the contrary of most other disorders which are increasingly related to YLDs in later life [8, 9]. According to the 2019 GBS study, migraine was considered as the second major motive leading to disability in the world and the first among young women [5].

Migraine impacts both the direct costs related to healthcare benefits and the indirect costs associated with absenteeism from work, decreased productivity as well as the other intangible conditions, such as the time spent on trying to find appropriate care or the time taken away from patient's own family tasks [10]. A large European study has demonstrated that migraine has quite high personal impact and that 17.7% of males and 28.0% of females with migraine have lost over 10 days of activities during a 3-month period [11]. The Eurolight study has exhibited an estimation of an annual cost of headache at €173 million, and €111 million (64%) imputed to migraine of which direct expenditures have been accounted for 7% and indirect costs for 93%. Direct health-care costs related to migraine have been found to be €1222 per person in Europe [12]. The International Burden of Migraine Study (IBMS) has found an estimation of individual annual cost of €793.22 for episodic and €2422.11 for chronic migraine with pertinent differentiation detected across countries [7]. The cost of attack-associated productivity loss is considered as the most significant factor of financial concern related to headache disorders, which has been calculated to account for 79–93% of total costs of headache. Work productivity has been found to influence 54.3% of the workers in a large sample of a dynamic labour force during a headache attack. The estimated annual indirect costs of headache has been determined to be up to €664.88 per worker with headache disorder [13].

Taking into account these widespread consequences of headache, it is significant to evaluate headahe-related disability such as the headache impact on patients' life and activities [14]. The first tool to measure the disability in patients with headache is the Headache Disability Inventory (HDI) developed by Jacobson et al. in 1994 [14]. Ever since, many patient-reported outcome measures (PROMs) providing an unbiased methodology of a subjective construct have been developed for evaluating the perceptions of personal functioning and wellbeing of the headache patients during or between the attacks to measure the headache impact and disability such as the Migraine Disability Assessment (MIDAS) and Headache Impact Test (HIT-6) [15–18]. The purpose, number of items, and recall period of the clinical instruments for disability, impact and burden in headache and migraine are presented in Table 7.1.

**Table 7.1** The purpose, number of items and recall period of the instruments

| Instrument | Purpose | Item | Recall period |
|---|---|---|---|
| MIGSEV | Measure the severity of migraine | 7 | |
| HImQ | Measure the pain intensity and limitations of activity from headache | 8 | 3 months |
| MIDAS | Measure the disability caused by migraine on paid labour, household chores and other daily activities | 5 | 3 months |
| HALT Index | Measure the headache disability | 5 | 3 months for HALT-90<br>1 month for HALT-30<br>1 week for HALT-7 |
| HIT | Measure the impact of headache on functional health and well-being | 6 | 1 month for the last three questions but no recall period for the first three questions |
| FAIM | Measure functional status associated with migraine | 14 | |
| HANA | Measure two dimensions of the chronic effect of migraine (frequency and bothersomeness) | 7 | 1 month |
| MIBS-4 | Measure the migraine-related burden in-between migraine attacks (interictal period) | 4 | 1 month |
| HDI | Measure headache disability | 25 | |
| HADLI | Measure the disability associated with headache focusing merely on substantial daily life activities | 9 | 1 month |
| BURMIG | Measure the burden of migraine | 77 | 3 months |
| EUROLIGHT | Measure the personal, social and economic impact of primary headache disorders | 103 | 3 months<br>1 day for questions regarding yesterday |
| HARDSHIP | Measure the headache-attributed burden | 101 | 3 months for burden questions<br>1 day for questions of 'headache yesterday' |
| MPFID | Measure the migraine impacts on physical functioning and social interactions | 13 | 1 day |
| MFIQ | Measure the impact of migraine on physical, social, and emotional functioning | 26 | 1 week |
| MWPLQ | Measure the impact of migraine on hours missed from work and impaired productivity while at work | 29 | Most recent episode |
| HEADWORK | Measure the migraine induced work-associated disability | 17 | 1 month |

*MIGSEV* migraine severity scale, *HImQ* headache impact questionnaire, *MIDAS* migraine disability assessment scale, *HALT* headache-attributed lost time, *HIT* headache impact test, *FAIM* functional assessment in migraine, *HANA* headache needs assessment, *MIBS-4* migraine interictal burden scale-4, *HDI* Henry Ford Hospital headache disability inventory, *HADLI* headache activity of daily living index, *BURMIG* burden of migraine instrument, *HARDSHIP* headache-attributed restriction, disability, social handicap, and impaired participation, *MPFID* migraine physical function impact diary, *MFIQ* migraine functional impact questionnaire, *MWPLQ* migraine work and productivity loss questionnaire

Disability measurement of the patients with headache disorders can predict the intensity of disease and influences of headache on functional status and on the psychosocial and financial aspects of life. PROMs provides physicians to adjust headache treatment plans in line with the severity of disease, to track the response to therapy over time, helps to improve the outcomes, and result in significant improvements in patients' lives [19]. They may also facilitate communication between a physician and a patient paving the way for monitoring the disability in the community [16]. There are different methods of interpretation change scores resulting from PROMs. The within-person minimal important change (MIC) is "the smallest change in score over time that a patient considers as important". Between-group 'minimally important difference' (MID) is another method for researchers to interpret differences between two groups of patients [20]. In this article, we present a review of clinical instruments for disability, impact and burden in headache and migraine.

### 7.1.1  The Migraine Severity Scale (MIGSEV)

MIGSEV, a seven-item questionnaire, has been developed as a simple scale to assess the severity of migraine attacks [21]. The scale has consisted of three dimensions: intensity of attacks, frequency of attacks, and resistance to treatment. The questions have measured the attack-span and frequency, headache induced pain, incompetency while performing daily activities, presence of nausea or vomiting, and resistance to treatment and tolerability of treatment, which could be rated on a three- or four-point scale individually. Migraine attacks have been categorized as mild, moderate or severe. Seven items measuring severity have been composed by way of reviewing literature, consensus of expert neurologist, and patient inteviews. Analysis of main components has determined three dimensions giving an account of 65% of the all variance associated with intensity of attacks, frequency of attacks, and resistance to treatment. The validation of MIGSEV has been performed in a pilot study of 287 migraineurs and supported by good correlation between the severity items and a migraine-specific quality of life instrument (QVM; Quality de Vie en Migraine). It has shown substantive measurement properties in terms of reliability, reproducibility and sensitivity. Cronbach's a coefficient for the MIGSEV scale is 0.84 for physician assessment and 0.86 for patient assessment. Test-retest reliability of MIGSEV is strong ($\kappa 0 0.60$–0.71).

### 7.1.2  The Headache Impact Questionnaire (HImQ)

HImQ, an eight-item self-applied instrument, has measured the pain intensity and limitations of activity from headache over a 3-month span [22]. The HImQ has included 16 questions regarding the total number of headaches in the previous

3 months, headache duration, last headache, pain intensity (two questions), need for bed rest (two questions), incapacity while performing certain domains of activity (seven questions about interference with ability to work, handling household chores, and being engaged in non-work activity), and symptoms (two questions). The HImQ score has been calculated from eight items and represented the sum of average pain intensity (on a scale of 0–10) and total number of lost days with regards to work outside the home, household chores, and pastime activities. Decreased efficiency day equivalents have been also taken into account. HImQ has exhibited good internal consistency. Cronbach's alpha has been found to be 0.83. The test-retest reliability has been relatively high (average Pearson's r = 0.86). Moreover, eight-item HImQ scores have been compared with a 90-day daily diary measuring lost time in each of the domains assessed by HImQ and the HImQ score has found to be moderately valid (average Pearson's r = 0.49) [23]. Moderate to high convergent validity with the expert physician judgment of disability has been detected. The highest convergent validity has been found for frequency-based items. The major constraint of HImQ is the intricacy of scoring as it requires several calculations such as multiplication and addition [24].

### 7.1.3   Migraine Disability Assessment Scale (MIDAS)

A short five-item individually applied questionnaire MIDAS is the most frequently used disability scale to quantify disability caused by migraine over the preceding 3 months [17]. It has been developed by Stewart and et al. on the basis of HImQ [25]. The effect of migraine on day-to-day activities has been evaluated from a three-perspective approach through five questions. The first and second questions have been directed towards paid or school work, the third and fourth questions for household chores, and the last question for nonwork related time (pastime and social gatherings). The two questions for each of the first two groups (paid work/ schoolwork, household work) were asked to inquire about the number of days of missed activity or days in which the efficiency has been decreased by at least half as a result of headache [26]. These dimensions have been chosen due to their sigificance to people between the ages of 20 and 50 who have the highest prevalence of headache [25]. Additional two questions (A and B) have inquired headache frequency (number of days with migraine in the previous 3 months) and pain severity (average pain severity of headache attacks) in a 0 (no pain at all) to 10 (pain as bad as it could be) scale. These additional questions are not included in the calculation.

The MIDAS lacks complexity to apply and assess the outcome. The scale takes a few minutes to apply. The score has derived as the sum of scores (number of days affected) of the first five questions. Consequently, the score has owned units of lost days. The maximum MIDAS score per day is 3 and the maximum score for 3 months is 270, as each day of the headache can lead to loss-time when performing an activity mentioned in each of these three domains. Total scores are to be interpreted both as a continuous variable as well as a factor assigning respondents to one of four disability grades: grade I, little or no disability (score of 0–5); grade II, mild disability (score of 6–10); grade III, moderate disability (score of 11–20); and grade IV, severe disability (score of 21). Furthernore, the severe disability grade (grade IV) is divided into two grades as grade IV-A, severe disability (scores of 21–40) and grade IV-B, very severe disability (scores of 41–270) to provide for greater benefit for the most common and severe headache disorders (eg, chronic migraine) [17].

There has been widespread proof for reliability and validity of the MIDAS. Psychometric evaluation of MIDAS has been conducted in two different studies. The MIDAS assessment has included the participants both with migraine headache and with nonmigraine headache and the result of the aforementioned assessment has revealed that the participants with migraine significantly expressed more concern on the missed days in all three domains of activities ($P < 0.001$). Moreover, participants with migraine have noticed significantly more days in which their productivity has gone down for paid tasks and household chores ($P < 0.001$). The test-retest Spearman's correlations of items have varried between 0.67 and 0.73. Spearman's correlation for the MIDAS score has been found to be 0.84. Cronbach's alpha for internal consistency has been determined to be 0.83 [25]. MIDAS has been also validated against a 90 day daily diary recording daily time loss in each of the three dimensions evaluated by MIDAS in a study incorporating 144 participants with migraine [27]. Participants have been requested to provide orderly diary entries being a record of their migraine and observation of productivity during the 3-month period of study and to fulfill the MIDAS presented in the last stage of the study. Spearman's correlation coefficients between the items of MIDAS and composite diary results have ranged from 0.41 to a high of 0.76. Association between diary and the MIDAS has been found to be relatively high for average pain intensity and number of days with headache. MIDAS has been found to be fairly correlated with diary summary scores (Spearman's r = 0.63). MIDAS scores have been immensely associated with decisions of physicians about the requirements for treatment.

For MIDAS, no MID has been established [28]. MIC for MIDAS after nonpharmacological treatment has been determined to be 4.5 points [29].

A variant of MIDAS has been developed for assessing the impact of migraines in pediatric patients (PedMIDAS) [30]. It has been translated and validated into many languages [17]. Recently, a minor change has been made in the original MIDAS questionnaire for reducing recall bias and improving precision of the results. The recall period has been changed from 3 months to 4 weeks and the questionnaire has named as mMIDAS [31].

The questionnaire has been widely applied in migraine clinical practice and trials. It is a considerable component of a combination of academical, investigative, and therapeutical measurements and can perform a crucial part to improve the lives of migraine patients as well as the ones suffering from other headache types. It has been denoted that the grade of MIDAS has provided a base for choosing initial treatment in stratified care. MIDAS has evaluated both entirely lost days as well as the substantially (>50%) decreased activity because of headace. This is significant because previous studies have shown that patients with headaches frequently resume their usual activities but with decreased efficiency during therir attacks [26]. This question format has presented a significant advantage over the HImQ as it has provided a simple way to obtain a disability score in easily interpretable units.

There has been some limitations of MIDAS questionnaire. The tool has measured disability only during attacks but not in-between the attacks. It has also missed the burden imposed during the attacks that does not lead to considerable decrease of activity. It has assessed what people prefer to do rather than what they can do. There has been the problem of ceiling effect with excessively frequent and burdensome headache although an additional cut score has been developed for chronic migraine. Furthermore, it has not been officially validated for other headache disorders [17, 24].

### 7.1.4 Headache-Attributed Lost Time (HALT) Index

HALT Index, a direct and close derivative of MIDAS, has been developed by Lifting The Burden [32]. HALT has provided an evaluation of headache disability, its primary outcome of lost productive time and the secondary burden of financial cost. HALT consists of five questions. Questions 1 and 2 are asked to unveil lost productive time (entirely lost days) (absenteeism) and days of <50% productivity (presenteeism) from work related to headache. Work might be defined as an employee with regular income or a freelancer. For children, it implies school related tasks. Questions 3 and 4 evaluate the household chores. "Household chores" refers to the range of tasks performed daily at home. Although its nature might be gender-related to some extent, "household work" is not restricted to the chores associated to women in many cultures. Question 5 is closely related to the days of missed social event due to headache.

The original form of HALT is HALT-90 which has recorded days affected by headache preceding 3 months (90 days) period. HALT-30 and HALT-7/30 are alternative versions. HALT-30 has measured the headache burden of each individual over 1 month (30 days) as shorter period can provide reducing recall error problems. This version has been well shown in the special setting of a workplace-based clinic in Turkey, where HALT-30 has been used in base-line evaluations to determine treatment priority [33]. HALT-7/30, a variant of HALT-30, has inquiried only lost work days in the preceding month (30 days) and week (7 days) for population-based studies of the burden attributable to headache, including financial cost.

It is easy to analyze and score like MIDAS. In order to assess total lost productive time from work, days wholly lost through absenteeism have been added to days of presenteeism with <50% productivity because of headache; by way of counterbalance, headache-influenced days have been disregarded in which the productivity was still more than 50%. Lost household work time has been calculated in the same way. For avoiding double-counting, an instruction has been given (on a single day, productivity both at work and in the housework performance might decrease more than 50%). Total lost productive time is the sum of lost work time and lost household work time from the first four questions. Question 5, on the other hand, has led to an uncomplicated calculation for which the unit is not whole days. When this count has been added to any of these scores, a mistake has occured. Moreover, adding question 5 in a sum of answers has also caused double counting when a day lost at work has been followed by a lost social event in the same evening. Nonetheless, the counting of missed social occurrence has stated the additional burden, therefore question 5 has been kept in HALT-90 and counted in the total summed score (summation of all five questions), leading grading. Grade I, minimal or infrequent impact (days lost in last 3 months of 0–5); grade II, mild or infrequent impact (days lost in last 3 months of 6–10); grade III, moderate impact (days lost in last 3 months of 11–20); grade IV, severe impact (days lost in last 3 months of $\geq$20). Grading is valuable to point out the level of a patient's private necessity and, maybe, a priority for therapy. HALT-30 and HALT-7/30 do not incorparate grading.

HALT index can be easily used in all headache disorders [34]. It is freely used for clinical, research or other academic purposes [32]. There has been no separately validation for clinical settings until now, but applied in epidemiological studies in various countries and languages. One of the limitations of the questionnaire is that it has evaluated only ictal burden [24].

## 7.1.5   Headache Impact Test (HIT)

HIT has been firstly programmed as a computerized adaptative questionnaire to measure the impact of headache. There has been evidence of it to be precise, reliable, valid, and clinically relevant in assessment [35, 36]. Afterwards, the six-item Headache Impact Test (HIT-6) based on the Internet-HIT question pool, a short paper and pencil form of HIT, has been designed to globally assess the impact of headache on the competency to function in a normal manner in daily life [18]. HIT-6 items have been selected from the 54 ones of existing adverse headache impact item pool and from 35 items recommended by clinicians. These six items evaluate negative headache impact on pain intensity, common daily activities including household work, job-related, school or social activities, wish to lie down when a patient suffers from headache, fatigue, frustration, and difficulty in concentrating. The last three questions focus on headache over the preceding 4 weeks but no recall period has been pointed out for the first three questions. The patient has replied each question using five answer categories: never, rarely, sometimes, very often, or always. Each category has been related to a specific number of points (6, 8, 10, 11, and 13 points, respectively). Total HIT-6 score has been obtained by addition of these responses, in a range of 36–78 with higher scores indicating very severe impact on the daily respondent's life. Scores $\leq$49 have indicated little to no impact on life; 50–55 have indicated some impact on life; 56–59 have indicated considerable impact on life; and $\geq$ 60 have indicated very severe impact on life. Scores can be interpreted using four groupings indicating the headache impact severity on the patient's life [18, 35, 36].

The evidence has demonstrated the HIT-6 to be psychometrically sound and clinically relevant. Internal consistency, alternate forms, and test-retest reliability of the HIT-6 have been found to be well with coefficients of 0.89, 0.90, and 0.80, respectively. HIT-6 has shown good discriminant validity and robust capability for discriminating between the headache diagnosis and severity with relative validity coefficients of 0.82 and 1.00. Moreover, the HIT-6 is proved to be perfectly convenient in terms of access and use. The instrument can be applied and scored in 2–3 min, that is suitable within the typical consultation time interval in general practice. Therefore, HIT-6 has differentiated from other measurements of paper-based headache effect by combining precision with shortness, features which make it ideal for using in busy clinical practices [18]. Since the initial development and validation of HIT-6, it has been acknowledged and extensively used in clinical practice, and implemented to clinical trials or observational studies for using in screening and monitoring of treatment in patients with headaches with the inclusion of migraine. The between-group MID for HIT-6 in has been reported to be a decrease of at least 2.3 points for chronic migraine [37] and 1.5 points for episodic migraine [20]. The within-patient MID for HIT-6 has been reported to be ≥5.0 points decrease [38]. The within-person MIC has been estimated to be between 2.5 and 6 points [20]. Translations and validations of HIT-6 exist in multiple languages [24].

The limitations of HIT-6 are that it is scored in optional units, multiplication is required for scoring, has ceiling and floor effect problems, and has copyrights [24].

### 7.1.6 Functional Assessment in Migraine (FAIM) Questionnaire

FAIM, migraine-spesific self-administered questionnare, has been derived from the International Classification of Impairments, Disabilities, and Handicaps, version 2 classification system devised by the World Health Organization (WHO). The instrument measures functional status associated with migraine, that has contained three dimensions as follows mental functioning, activity and participation [39]. The instrument has covered nine Mental Functioning items assessing domains of Attention/Thought (five items) and Perception (four items), and a list of 28 Activity and Participation items from which patients have chosen five elements most pertinent to their habits and daily conducts. Construct validity has been analyzed with correlating three FAIM aspects featuring Role Restrictive, Role Preventive, Emotional Function of Migraine-Specific Quality of Life (MSQoL) questionnare and dimensions of Mental Functioning and Physical Functioning of Short form Health Survey (SF-12). There has been no significant correlations between FAIM and dimensions of SF-12. Moderately significant correlation has been found between the FAIM and MSQoL. The correlation between FAIM and the Emotional dimension of the MSQoL questionnare has been determined to be the lowest. No significant correlation has been detected with SF-12 component scores. Construct validity has also been assessesed through the comparison of results of each FAIM dimension with self-reported assessments of symptom severity and functional impairment. FAIM dimensions have been found significantly correlated with symptom severity in a positive manner and negatively correlated with functional status. Cronbach's α values have been found to be higher than 0.70 for all items of Mental Functioning. The reliability test has not been analyzed for the FAIM.

Researchers performing clinical evaluation with functional evaluation can skip the items of Perception elements applying a shorter tool.

### 7.1.7 The Headache Needs Assessment (HANA) Survey

HANA, seven-item brief and self-applied tool has been devised to measure two dimensions of the chronic effect of migraine (frequency and bothersomeness). The tool has probed seven issues to assess frequency and bothersomeness associated with living with migraine: anxiety/worry, depression/discouragement, self-control, energy, function/work, family/social activities, and overall impact [40].

Developers have performed validation studies through a Web-based survey, a clinical trial responsiveness population, and a retest reliability population. They have applied characteristics of headache such as frequency, severity, and treatment, demographic information, and the HDI for external validation. Floor or ceiling effects are yet to be determined. This instrument has fulfilled the standards for validity with good internal consistency, reliability, construct validity, and responsiveness. It has shown good test-retest reliability (Pearson's r = 0.77) and internal consistency (Cronbach's alpha 0.92, eigenvalue for the single factor 4.8). External validity has demonstrated that HANA scores have been statistically significantly correlated with HDI scores (0.73, $P < 0.0001$) and highly correlated with headache and treatment characteristics. HANA scores have deteriorated with higher scores of disability. Aforementioned affirmative correlations between the HANA total score and headache and treatment characteristics have pointed out that the HANA can distinguish less severe and more severe headache types and determine changes after medication.

HANA is proved to be a useful screening instrument to identify the problems. It can be applied to other headache disorders. Comparison between the HANA scores before treatment and after treatment can be performed to define the impact. Primary care providers can use the HANA to screen migraine patients with an aim to lead a more thorough assessment. Once defined, severe migraine patients might be subject to a prompt therapy with pain-relieving or preventive medications.

The HANA offers several advantages. For physicians, choosing promptly the suitable treatment decreases the number of visits. For employers, days lost from work and decrease in efficiency due to insufficient headache treatment can get reduced. For patients, it offers the opportunity of early recognition and treatment without the ordinary slow progression through stepped-care algorithms.

### *7.1.8   The Migraine Interictal Burden Scale (MIBS-4)*

MIBS-4, brief four-item self administered instrument, has been designed to measure the migraine-related burden in-between migraine attacks (interictal period) for clinical or research use. The four items have evaluated impairment at work or school, disruption in family and social life, difficulty in making plans or commitments, and emotional/affective and cognitive distress [41]. This instrument has specifically inquired the migraine effect over the preceding 4 weeks on days without migraine attack. The items are rated on a five-point scale: don't know/not applicable, never, rarely, some of the time, much of the time, or most or all of the time. A total score representing one of the four levels of interictal burden has been obtained by multiplying the answers to each question, ranging from 0 to 12. Greater scores have shown more iterictal burden classified as four levels: none (score of 0), mild (score of 1–2), moderate (score of 3–4), and severe (score 5). Each category provides advice on treatment [41, 42].

The development of this scale originated in a large survey-based study with 30 candidate questions determined from available outcome measures and focus groups. Then, psychometric validation was made to decrease the number of questions and evalute the reliability and validity in a population sample. MIBS-4 has been psychometrically tested and validated in a survey mailed to a sample of 2500 individuals with headache. Test-retest reliability has been found high across all retest intervals (rho = 0.69). MIBS-4 has been moderately positively correlated with MIDAS (Spearman's r = 0.40), HIT-6 (Spearman's r = 0.44), depression (Spearman's r = 0.41), absenteeism (Spearman's r = 0.18), and presenteeism (Spearman's r = 0.25). The moderate positive asociation detected between MIBS-4 and MIDAS has been put forward that ictal burden only partially predicts interictal burden. As anticipated, the MIBS-4 has been moderately correlated with MSQ in a negative manner (total score (r = −0.48) and subscales), meaning that as interical burden increases quality of life reduces [41, 42].

There has been no validation of the MIBS-4 for conditions other than migraine. This scale is less useful for patients with frequent headaches where interictal terms are limited or sparce [24].

### *7.1.9   The Henry Ford Hospital Headache Disability Inventory (HDI)*

HDI is one of the most exhaustive instrument which has been designed to measure headache disability. It has been developed to assess the headache impact on functional as well as emotional aspects of everyday life. The Alpha version of HDI (α-HDI) includes 40 items, each requesting "yes" (four points), "sometimes" (two points), or "no" (zero points) answers. These items have been derived from responses reflecting the history of headache patients in the trial. From the α-HDI, Jacobson et al. have derived a self-administered 25-item beta version (β-HDI) that has two domains offering emotional (13 items) and functional (12 items) impairment [14]. The questionnaire has a paper-based format. Instructions are provided at the beginning of the scale. The patients reply each item using three answer options: "yes" (four points), "sometimes" (two points), or "no" (0 points). Summation of scores determines the disability level. In this instrument, the maximum and minimum obtainable scores are 100 and 0, respectively, which can be converted to a total percent score of 100. The maximum obtainable scores for the functional and emotional subscales are 48 and 52, respectively. A maximum score of 100 points indicates the highest level of headache disability [38]. For total percent; 10–28% has denoted mild disability; 30–48% moderate disability; 50–68% severe disability; and > 70% complete disability.

The HDI has shown high internal consistency, good content validity, and strong test-retest reliability for long-term (2 month) (Pearson's r = 0.83) and short-term (1 week) (Pearson's r = 0.93). 95% confidence interval for test-retest change has been found to be 15.81 points for the total score. A 16-point change in total score might be presumed to reflect a true change in self-perceived headache disability (at the $P < 0.05$ level). It has shown high convergent validity (Pearson's r = 0.78) with the patients spouse's perception, as evaluated with the Spouse HDI. The spouse tool is same to the HDI with the exception that the word "I" displaces with the words "my spouse" in most cases. Also, high convergent validity with migraine severity but low convergent validity with HANA has been detected [43]. Furthermore, the validity and reliability of HDI in non-English verisons have been confirmed [44, 45].

The completion of this generic headache disability scale is easy. The scoring and interpreting of it is also simple. The HDI has been broadly used in the associated research studies [15, 46, 47]. It has evaluated different medical and rehabilitation treatment effects on the disabilities of physical and emotional aspects in patients with different headaches types, measured both ictal and interictal headache burden, and can be used to compare different disability aspects for various headache disorders [14].

### 7.1.10  *Headache Activity of Daily Living Index (HADLI)*

HADLI has been effectuated by significantly modifying the Neck Disability Index. It has been developed to measure the disability associated with headache focusing merely on substantial daily life activities [15]. This self-reported instrument has one domain comprising of nine items: Personal care, Lifting, Reading (including computers), Sleeping (over last week), Exercising (over last week), Social Activities,

Work, Driving or Travelling, Recreation. Instructions at the top of the tool have pointed out that the period for self-rating is within 1 month. Respondents are required to reply the each item according to instruction of "when I have a headache"in order to more exactly determine the context for self-rating The respondents have options of six-point categorical answer, where 0 is best ability and 5 is the worst. The total score of HADLI ranges from 0 to 45 with the highest score indicating maximum activity disability, which is converted to a percent score of 0–100. This scale can be completed in an average of 3 min.

The patients attending a private pain rehabilitation clinic and a chiropractic clinic due to migraine, tension-type, or cervicogenic headaches have constituted the study sample of HADLI. The participants have been collected by advertisement and personal demand. No floor or ceiling effects for total score has been detected. Face validity has been evaluated by focus group input and first-level psychometrics. The total Index Cronbach $\alpha$ has been found to be 0.96. The Principal Components Analysis have determined one component that accounted for 75% of the variance. This component has been termed activity disability. The correlation between the component of activity based disability and the total score of HADLI has been stated to be 0.99. The HADLI has shown good face validity but its psychometric properties are yet to be comprehensively assessed (450).

### 7.1.11   Burden of Migraine Instrument (BURMIG)

BURMIG, a self-reported questionnaire, has been developed to measure the burden of migraine, containing headache characteristics, disability due to migraine, comorbidities, management, and the impacts on the patients' lives [48]. The instrument includes 77 items out of 17% are open ended inquires. Biographical details have been provided the respondents. For the diagnosis of migraine, 'ID migraine' questions have been included. Specific parameters on headache as onset age, the average number of days with headache per month over the preceding 3 months, and symptoms before and after the headaches, information on general health, preceding and present disorders through the use of items from the World Health Organization Disability Assessment Schedule II (WHODAS II), MIDAS and the Patient Health Questionnaire-9 (PHQ-9) have been collected. Respondents have been asked to provide information on the effect of headaches on their professional and private life; their experience of consultation to physicians as well as the diagnosis made and medicine prescribed. Psychosocial conditions that worsen the headaches, impairment in social activities, headache conceptions and the requirement for support from health care professionals to ameliorate the headaches have been evaluated.

This instrument has been tested in 130 patients with headache (20 pain clinic, 17 primary care and 93 lay organisations) in Luxembourg which has been chosen as the country to perform the multicultural test run for the validation. BURMIG has shown strong reliability test. Retest-reliability for the diverse sections of the instrument has ranged between 0.6 and 1.0 (Kappa coefficient), with an intracorrelation coefficient of 0.7–1.0. The item 'Feeling tired or having little energy' from PHQ9 has demonstrated little re-test reliability at 1 month period. Internal consistency has been obtained to be acceptable for the MIDAS and somewhat smaller for items from WHODASII and PHQ9, which has been between 0.74 and 0.91 (Cronbach's alpha). Acceptable construct validity has been determined when samples have been adequately selected to discriminate between the headache levels. On the other hand, a poor discrimination between headache patients and the general population has been found in questions from WHODAS. Concerning the management of disease, Kappa coefficient has been between 0.68 and 1.00 which represents good agreement between the two steps. BURMIG has been translated into four languages (German, French, Portuguese, and English). The application of the aforementioned instrument is cumbersome.

## 7.1.12   *EUROLIGHT Questionnaire*

EUROLIGHT questionnaire has been developed to collect information on the personal, social and economic impact of primary headache disorders in Europe [49]. It has been taken as a basis in large from the BURMIG questionnaire, and additional items were gathered from the tools developed by Lifting The Burden. EUROLIGHT questionnaire has included 103 items, 7% of which are open questions, 15% numerical questions and 78% categorical. It has multiple parts. The first part is about demographic information (age, gender) and social situation (occupation, marital status, income, educational level, language). The upcoming part entails screening questions for headache (life-time and 1-year prevalence), followed by chronic daily headache questions. The next questions are for diagnosing the headache which the respondents consider to be the most bothersome (if the patient identifies more than one type of headache). The headache diagnostic questions have been based on the criteria of the International Classification of Headache Disorders, second edition (ICHD-II). The following questions are concerned with age at onset and headache frequency over the preceding 3 months. This section is followed by inquiries concerning headache of the previous day (duration, severity, influence, medication), and then by parts on the usage of health care resources containing such as medications, diagnostic investigations, hospital admission and the headache impact questions with regards to job, family life and social activities (with the inclusion of the HALT Index), for the patients with headache as well as for their household. Body mass index (BMI) questions have been asked as higher BMI might be a substantial and potentially curable risk factor for frequent headache. At last of the questionnaire, there are questions highlighting the level of quality of life (WHOQoL) in addition to the depression and anxiety related inquiries (Hospital Anxiety and Depression Scale). Filling of EUROLIGHT questionnaire takes almost 15–20 min.

This questionnaire has been validated in in five languages with 426 participants (131 in UK, 107 in Spain, 83 in Germany/Austria, 60 in Italy, and 45 in France). The rates of response have been varried between 73 and 100% in the different countries. It has demonstrated acceptable construct validity, excellent internal consistency, and good reliability test. Test–retest reliability has been ranged from −0.27 to 1.0. The internal consistency has been found to be range of 0.69–0.91.

### 7.1.13 Headache-Attributed Restriction, Disability, Social Handicap and Impaired Participation (HARDSHIP) Questionnaire

Global Campaign against Headache have developed guidelines for population-based studies of the headache-attributed burden [32, 50]. As a result of this campaign, a questionnaire assessing the headache-attributed restriction, disability, social handicap and impaired participation has been devised and termed HARDSHIP.

HARDSHIP questionnaire has been designed for administration by trained lay interviewers. This instrument consists of a modular design, in which separate sets of question have included demographic features, screening for headache caseness (presence or absence of headache disorder, ever and in the preceding year), diagnosing the type of headache and addressing each of the various quantifiable headacahe-related burden components including symptom burden; usage of health-care resource; disability and losses in productive time using the HALT index; influence on education, career and income; perception of control; interictal burden; overall individual burden (as willingness to pay for efficient treatment); effects on relationships and family dynamics; effects on other people including household members and children; quality of life using WHOQoL-8 question set; subjective wellbeing questions taken from the UK-ONS 2012 survey; comorbidity with the inclusion of obesity. Diagnostic questions for migraine, TTH, and medication overuse headache have based on the criteria of the International Classification of Headache Disorders, third edition beta version (ICHD-3 beta). Patients with more than one headache type have been required to focus on the most bothersome headache for ensuring that they have answered the questions with only one type of headache in mind. The instrument can identify the patients with headache on ≥15 days/month, and reveal possible medication overuse.

HARDSHIP questionnaire is translated into multiple languages and used in many geographical locations. It has been validated against the diagnoses of headache experts in numerous different settings. The diagnostic question set has been shown relatively insensitivity for TTH in all tested languages and cultures [51].

### 7.1.14   Migraine Physical Function Impact Diary (MPFID)

MPFID, a novel self-administered instrument, has been designed to measure the migraine impacts on physical functioning, including physical ability, difficulty moving the head or body, ability to conduct everyday activities, and impact on social interactions over the past 24 h following 2009 US Food and Drug Administration (FDA) guidance on development of PROs for inclusion in clinical trials to support labeling claims [52, 53]. This instrument has been developed based on concept elicitation interviews. Cognitive interviews have been administered to further investigate content validity. The preliminary version of the instrument has 17 items in three dimensions stating the impact on daily activities, overall influence on every day activities, and physical impairment. By removing 4 items, a 13-item MPFID (version 2.0) form has been created, which includes domain of Impact on Everyday Activities containing seven items, domain of the Physical Impairment containing five items, and one stand-alone global item providing an evaluation of the overall impact of migraine on everyday activities (Item 9). 24-h recall period has been chosen to prevent recall bias. The patients have options of five-point categorical response with items of difficulty varying between 'without any difficulty' and 'unable to do' and with items of frequency varying between 'none of the time' and 'all of the time', with five indicating the greatest burden. The scores for each domain have been calculated with summation of the responses of each item. The total score has ranged from 0 to 100 with higher scores defining higher burden.

This instrument has exhibited strong psychometric properties [54]. The domains of everyday activities and physical impairments have been demonstrated high internal consistency (Cronbach alpha = 0.97 and 0.93) and good test–retest reliability in a large sample of subjects with episodic migraine and cronic migraine (intraclass correlations coefficient = 0.74 and 0.77). Convergent validity has been exhibited by moderate associations between the scores of MPFID domain and number of migraine days, headache days, bed days, and other PRO instruments containing HIT-6, Patient Reported Outcomes Measurement Information System Physical Function Short Form 10a (PROMIS-PF), Migraine-Specific Quality of Life Questionnaire (MSQ; version 2.1), Patient Global Rating of Change, and Patient Global Impression of Severity (r = ±0.50–0.68; $P < 0.0001$). The scores of Everyday Activities and Physical Impairments have been found to able to differentiate between the groups of subjects with clinically diverse headache variables and scores of other PROs instrument ($P < 0.05$). Evidence has been provided through the use of MPFID for assessing functional outcomes of interventions for migraine in clinical trial and practice. The MPFID allows the assessment of the effects of migraine on ictal days and interictal days. In the United States, this instrument has been acknowledged as valid by the FDA and is inclusive of prescribing information for treatments of migraine.

### 7.1.15  The Migraine Functional Impact Questionnaire (MFIQ)

MFIQ, self-report questionnaire, has been designed to evaluate the impact of migraine on physical, social, and emotional functioning in the past 7 days [55]. It has been developed using methods compatible with the regulatory guidance on measures of PRO to support labeling claims regarding the treatments' benefit [53]. MFIQ has been proposed for usage in adult patients with episodic migraine or chronic migraine, with or without aura.

MFIQ (version 2) consists of 26 items, 4 domains named Physical Function (PF), Usual Activities (UA), Social Function (SF), and Emotional Function (EF), and global item named Overall Impact on UA. A 7-day recall period has been chosen in order to determine the week-to-week variability, which is a significant perspective of the frequent and episodic nature of migraine and naturally emerging fluctuations, and to decrease the potential recall bias related to longer recall period. The items of MFIQ have derived from the concept elicitation interviews with the patients and also content validity has been verified through cognitive interviews. Moreover, clinical experts in migraine have ensured input for developing and finalizing the questionnaire. Items have been used a five-point response scale. Total scores have ranged from 0 to 100, with higher scores pointing out greater impact.

MFIQ has robust psychometric properties [56]. All scores of the MFIQ have been demonstrated high internal consistency ($\alpha \geq 0.89$), moderate test-retest reliability among stable subjects (intraclass correlation coefficient $\geq 0.47$), and good convergent validity. Construct validity has been exhibited by significant associations (all $P < 0.0001$) between the scores of MFIQ domain, scores of associated PRO instruments (HIT-6, Patient-Reported Outcomes Measurement Information System Physical Function Short Form 10a, and MSQ), and the frequency of migraine days and headache days. All domain scores of the MFIQ have discriminated between subgroups defined based on established clinically severity levels, number of monthly migraine and headache days, scores of other PRO instruments, and migraine interference levels ($P < 0.05$). Improvements of MFIQ scores have been found to be in compliance with the improvement in clinical measures, in migraine interference with daily activities, in other PRO scores ($P < 0.05$), showing that this questionnaire has been responsive to changes in impact of migraine.

The MFIQ can be applied to measure and follow the migraine impact, assess therapeutic targets, determine gaps for intervention, and to improve communication between the healthcare providers and patients. It can also be applied to assess the outcome of migraine interventions in research and clinical practice settings. The translation and validation of MFIQ into 20 languages is handled.

### 7.1.16 Migraine Work and Productivity Loss Questionnaire (MWPLQ)

MWPLQ, a self-reported instrument, has been developed to assess the impact of migraine headache on capability of individual to do paid work in the past 24 h in line with MFIQ [57, 58]. Like MFIQ, it has been developed complying the methods defined in the guidance of FDA PRO. This questionnaire has collected the data about the number of hours of work lost due to migraine or treatment of migraine and the number of hours in which the productivity has diminished while at work. The data might be utilized to calculate the total number of hours of paid work lost because of migraine and to evaluate the time lost from work [59]. Furthermore, it incorporates the items on the treatment of migraine and questions associated with the most recent migraine attack. The MWPLQ consists of 29 items out of which 18 aim to reveal difficulty dealing with different tasks. These work difficulty questions have evaluated quality of work, quantity of work, interpersonal issues, management of time, bodily struggle, mental struggle, environmental triggers. There has been an additional question for whole impact on difficulty in working. Measurement of the items is calculated through the use of a six-point Likert scale in which the options have varried between 'no difficulty' and 'so much difficulty, couldn't do at all'. Moreover, the last question of the tool aims to shed light on the whole effectiveness of respondent on the job during the migraine headache. The respondent is expected to answer these questions by filling in percent, with 100% indicating the best and 0% indicating the worst. The application of the instrument takes about 20–25 min [57, 58].

The psychometric properties of this instrument have been evaluated with 265 patients with migraine in a 3-month clinical study. Participants have been requied to complete the MWPLQ following every migraine attack. The instrument has face validity. Cronbach's α has ranged between 0.80 and 0.95 for the domains of work difficulty, putting forward a high level of internal consistency. Work loss and domains of work difficulty have been moderately correlated with the severity of migraine and functional disability (r = 0.61–0.72). Correlation between MQoL and all measures associated with work has been found to be moderate to strong (−0.31, −0.65). The question of global work difficulty has been strongly correlated with the all domains of work difficulty (r > 0.70). The scores of SF-36 have been lowly to moderately correlated with work difficulty. On the whole, associations have supported construct validity of this tool. Also, the MWPLQ has been obviously distinguished between the patients receiving different types of migraine treatment over the study duration, with good discriminant validity [58].

### 7.1.17  *HEADWORK*

HEADWORK is a 17-item questionnaire, which has been designed to address the quantity and intensity of task-based challenges at work as well as the factors impacting on these challenges [60]. The developers have assessed prior literature reviews and focused on the episodic and chronic migraine patients for the purpose of developing a set of items to evaluate. The patients have been collected from eight Italian headache centers. The questionnare consists of two sections. The first part titled "Work-related difficulties" includes 11 factors evaluating the degree to which migraine headaches determine a difficulty in general skills such as paying attention to work tasks, problem solving or starting a new work task, or in specific tasks such as driving a car, using the computer or speaking and socializing with other people. The second section named "Factors Contributing to Work Difficulties" includes six items addressing the workplace's environmental triggers and attitudes of the co-workers. Responders have been asked to provide an answer using a five-point response scale ranging from 1 to 5. Items associated with work-related difficulties and factors that contributed to work difficulties have been explicated 67.1 and 52.1% of the total variance, respectively [61]. Both of the subcales of HEADWORK have shown good measurement properties, with higher scores being related to greater levels of impact. The scores of HEADWORK have been found to be higher in patients with chronic migraine for both scales in comparison with the patients with episodic migraine. The subscales of the HEADWORK have demonstrated that higher scores have been related to higher disability, lower quality of life, lower productivity, and higher frequency of headache and pain severity. Correlation indexes of the questionnaire have been detected higher with the WHODAS-12 than with the MSQ and with the MIDAS.

HEADWORK questionnaire can be efficiently used to evaluate the impact of triggers and treatments on work-related difficulties shedding light on cost-effectiveness of different treatments. It can be employed to address the work-related disability in epidemiological and clinical research studies assessing the episodic and chronic migraine burden.

## 7.2  Conclusion

There have been many self-report instruments developed to measure the impact, disability, and burden of the headache and migraine. These instruments can help to understand the intensity of disease and headache influences on functional, psychosocial and financial aspects of life. They provide physicians to adjust headache treatment plans according to severity of disease, enable to improve the outcomes, and all these contributions result in significant improvements in patients' lives.

# References


1. Milosevic N, Trajkovic JZ, Mijajlovic M, Milosevic J, Novakovic T, Vitosevic Z, et al. The burden and health care use of patients with migraine and tension-type headache in post-conflict area of Serbia. Cephalalgia. 2022;18:3331024221082061.
2. Saylor D, Steiner TJ. The global burden of headache. Semin Neurol. 2018;38(2):182–90.
3. Institute for Health Metrics and Evaluation. 2020. http://www.healthdata.org/results/gbd_summaries/2019/headache-disorders-level-3-cause
4. Steiner TJ, Stovner LJ, Jensen R, Uluduz D, Katsarava Z. Lifting the burden: the Global Campaign against Headache. Migraine remains second among the world's causes of disability, and first among young women: findings from GBD2019. J Headache Pain. 2020;21(1):137.
5. GBD 2019 Diseases and Injuries Collaborators. Global burden of 369 diseases and injuries in 204 countries and territories, 1990–2019: a systematic analysis for the Global Burden of Disease Study 2019. Lancet. 2020;396(10258):1204–22.
6. GBD 2016 Disease and Injury Incidence and Prevalence Collaborators. Global, regional, and national incidence, prevalence, and years lived with disability for 328 diseases and injuries for 195 countries, 1990–2016: a systematic analysis for the Global Burden of Disease Study 2016. Lancet. 2017;390(10100):1211–59.
7. Bloudek LM, Stokes M, Buse DC, Wilcox TK, Lipton RB, Goadsby PJ, et al. Cost of healthcare for patients with migraine in five European countries: results from the International Burden of Migraine Study (IBMS). J Headache Pain. 2012;13(5):361–78.
8. Vos T, Abajobir AA, Abate KH, et al. Global, regional, and national incidence, prevalence, and years lived with disability for 328 diseases and injuries for 195 countries, 1990–2016: a systematic analysis for the Global Burden of Disease Study 2016. Lancet. 2017;390:1211–59.
9. Stovner LJ, Nichols E, Steiner TJ, et al. Global, regional, and national burden of migraine and tension-type headache, 1990–2016: a systematic analysis for the Global Burden of Disease Study 2016. Lancet Neurol. 2018;17:954–76.
10. Leonardi M, Raggi A. A narrative review on the burden of migraine: when the burden is the impact on people's life. J Headache Pain. 2019;20(1):41.
11. Steiner TJ, Stovner LJ, Katsarava Z, Lainez JM, Lampl C, Lantéri-Minet M, et al. The impact of headache in Europe: principal results of the Eurolight project. J Headache Pain. 2014;15(1):31.
12. Linde M, Gustavsson A, Stovner LJ, Steiner TJ, Barré J, Katsarava Z, et al. The cost of headache disorders in Europe: the Eurolight project. Eur J Neurol. 2012;19(5):703–11.
13. Gil-Gouveia R, Miranda R. Indirect costs attributed to headache: a nation-wide survey of an active working population. Cephalalgia. 2022;42(4–5):317–25.
14. Jacobson GP, Ramadan NM, Aggarwal SK, Newman CW. The Henry Ford Hospital Headache Disability Inventory (HDI). Neurology. 1994;44:837–42.
15. Vernon H, Lawson G. Development of the headache activities of daily living index: initial validity study. J Manip Physiol Ther. 2015;38(2):102–11.
16. Houts CR, Wirth RJ, McGinley JS, Cady R, Lipton RB. Determining thresholds for meaningful change for the Headache Impact Test (HIT-6) total and item-specific scores in chronic migraine. Headache. 2020;60(9):2003–13.
17. Blumenfeld AM, Varon SF, Wilcox TK, Buse DC, Kawata AK, Manack A, et al. Disability, HRQoL and resource use among chronic and episodic migraineurs: results from the International Burden of Migraine Study (IBMS). Cephalalgia. 2011;31(3):301–15.
18. Kosinski M, Bayliss MS, Bjorner JB, Ware JE Jr, Garber WH, Batenhorst A, et al. A six-item short-form survey for measuring headache impact: the HIT-6. Qual Life Res. 2003;12(8):963–74.
19. Burch RC, Buse DC, Lipton RB. Migraine: epidemiology, burden, and comorbidity. Neurol Clin. 2019;37(4):631–49.
20. Smelt AF, Assendelft WJ, Terwee CB. What is a clinically relevant change on the HIT-6 questionnaire? An estimation in a primary-care population of migraine patients. Cephalalgia. 2014;34:29–36.

21. El Hasnaoui A, Vray M, Richard A, Nachit-Ouinekh F, Boureau F, MIGSEV Group. Assessing the severity of migraine: development of the MIGSEV scale. Headache. 2003;43:628–35.
22. Stewart WF, Lipton RB, Simon D, Von Korff M, Liberman J. Reliability of an illness severity measure for headache in a population sample of migraine sufferers. Cephalalgia. 1998;18:44–51.
23. Stewart WF, Lipton RB, Simon D, Libermana J, Korff MV. Validity of an illness severity measure for headache in a population sample of migraine sufferers. Pain. 1999;79:291–301.
24. Buse DC, Sollars CM, Steiner TJ, Jensen RH, Jumah MAA, Lipton RB. Why HURT? A review of clinical instruments for headache management. Curr Pain Headache Rep. 2012;16(3):237–54.
25. Stewart WF, Lipton RB, Kolodner K, Liberman J, Sawyer J. Reliability of the migraine disability assessment score in a population-based sample of headache sufferers. Cephalalgia. 1999;19(2):107–14.
26. Lipton RB, Stewart WF, Sawyer J, Edmeads JG. Clinical utility of an instrument assessing migraine disability: the Migraine Disability Assessment (MIDAS) questionnaire. Headache. 2001;41(9):854–61.
27. Stewart WF, Lipton RB, Kolodner KB, Sawyer J, Lee C, Liberman JN. Validity of the migraine disability assessment (MIDAS) score in comparison to a diary-based measure in a population sample of migraine sufferers. Pain. 2000;88:41–52.
28. Lipton R, Desai P, Sapra S, Buse D, Fanning K, Reed M. How much change in headache-related disability is clinically meaningful? Estimating minimally important difference (MID) or change in MIDAS using data from the AMPP Study [Abstract]. Boston: American Headache Society Annual Meeting; 2017.
29. Carvalho GF, Luedtke K, Braun T. Minimal important change and responsiveness of the Migraine Disability Assessment Score (MIDAS) questionnaire. J Headache Pain. 2021;22(1):126.
30. Hershey AD, Powers SW, Vockell AL, LeCates S, Kabbouche MA, Maynard MK. PedMIDAS: development of a questionnaire to assess disability of migraines in children. Neurology. 2001;57(11):2034–9.
31. Buse DC, Lipton RB, Hallström Y, Reuter U, Tepper SJ, Zhang F, Sapra S, Picard H, Mikol DD, Lenz RA. Migraine-related disability, impact, and health related quality of life among patients with episodic migraine receiving preventive treatment with Erenumab. Cephalalgia. 2018;38(10):1622–31.
32. Steiner TJ, World Headache Alliance. Lifting the burden: the global campaign against headache. Lancet Neurol. 2004;3(4):204–5.
33. Selekler HM, Gökmen G, Alvur TM, Steiner TJ. Productivity losses attributable to headache, and their attempted recovery, in a heavy-manufacturing workforce in Turkey: implications for employers and politicians. J Headache Pain. 2015;16:96.
34. Steiner TJ. The HALT and HART indices. J Headache Pain. 2007;8:S22–5.
35. Ware JE, Bjorner JB, Kosinski M. Practical implications of item response theory and computerized adaptive testing: a brief summary of ongoing studies of widely used headache impact scales. Med Care. 2000;38(Suppl II, 9):1173–82.
36. Bayliss MS, Dewey JE, Dunlap I, Batenhorst AS, Cady R, Diamond ML, et al. A study of the feasibility of internet administration of a computerized health survey: the headache impact test (HIT). Qual Life Res. 2003;12:953–61.
37. Coeytaux RR, Kaufman JS, Chao R, Mann JD, Devellis RF. Four methods of estimating the minimal important difference score were compared to establish a clinically significant change in Headache Impact Test. J Clin Epidemiol. 2006;59:374–80.
38. Yang M, Rendas-Baum R, Varon SF, Kosinski M. Validation of the headache impact test (HIT-6™) across episodic and chronic migraine. Cephalalgia. 2011;31:357–67.
39. Pathak DS, Chisolm DJ, Weis KA. Functional Assessment in Migraine (FAIM) questionnaire: development of an instrument based upon the WHO's International Classification of Functioning, Disability, and Health. Value Health. 2005;8:591–600.

40. Cramer JA, Silberstein SD, Winner P. Development and validation of the Headache Needs Assessment (HANA) survey. Headache. 2001;41:402–9.

41. Buse DC, Bigal MB, Rupnow M, Reed M, Serrano D, Lipton RB. Development and validation of the Migraine Interictal Burden Scale (MIBS): a self-administered instrument for measuring the burden of migraine between attacks [abstract S05.003]. Neurology. 2007;68(suppl 1):A89.

42. Buse D, Bigal M, Rupnow M, Reed LM. The Migraine Interictal Burden Scale (MIBS): results of a population-based validation study [abstract F64]. Headache. 2007;47(5):778.

43. Jacobson GP, Ramadan NM, Norris L, Newman CW. Headache disability inventory (HDI): short-term test-retest reliability and spouse perceptions. Headache. 1995;35(9):534–9.

44. Rodríguez-Franco L, Cano-García FJ, Blanco-Picabia I. Conductas de dolor y discapacidad en migrañas y cefaleas tensionales. Adaptación española del Pain Behavior Questionnaire (PBQ) y del headache disability inventory (HDI). Anál Modif Conducta. 2000;26(109):739–62.

45. Jabbari S, Salahzadeh Z, Sarbakhsh P, Rezaei M, Farhoudi M, Ghodrati M. Validity and Reliability of Persian Version of Henry Ford Hospital Headache Disability Inventory Questionnaire. Arch Iran Med. 2021;24(10):752–8.

46. Palacios-Ceña M, Castaldo M, Wang K, Catena A, Torelli P, Arendt-Nielsen L, et al. Relationship of active trigger points with related disability and anxiety in people with tension-type headache. Medicine (Baltimore). 2017;96(13):e6548.

47. John D, Ram D, Sundarmurthy H, Rathod H, Rathod S. Study of barrier to help seeking and its relationships with disability in patients with headache. J Clin Diagn Res. 2016;10(10):VC01–5.

48. Andrée C, Vaillant M, Rott C, Katsarava Z, Sándor PS. Development of a self reporting questionnaire, BURMIG, to evaluate the burden of migraine. J Headache Pain. 2008;9:309–15.

49. Andrée C, Vaillant M, Barre J, Katsarava Z, Lainez JM, Lair ML, et al. Development and validation of the EUROLIGHT questionnaire to evaluate the burden of primary headache disorders in Europe. Cephalalgia. 2010;30:1082–100.

50. Stovner LJ, Al Jumah M, Birbeck GL, Gururaj G, Jensen R, Katsarava Z, et al. The methodology of population surveys of headache prevalence, burden and cost: principles and recommendations from the Global Campaign against Headache. J Headache Pain. 2014;15(1):5.

51. Steiner TJ, Gururaj G, Andrée C, Katsarava Z, Ayzenberg I, Yu SY, et al. Diagnosis, prevalence estimation and burden measurement in population surveys of headache: presenting the HARDSHIP questionnaire. J Headache Pain. 2014;15(1):3.

52. Hareendran A, Mannix S, Skalicky A, Bayliss M, Blumenfeld A, Buse DC, et al. Development and exploration of the content validity of a patient-reported outcome measure to evaluate the impact of migraine- the migraine physical function impact diary (MPFID). Health Qual Life Outcomes. 2017;15(1):224.

53. Website. Food and Drug Administration. Guidance for industry patientreported outcome measures: use in medical product development to support labeling claims. FDA; 2009. http://www.fda.gov/downloads/Drugs/.../Guidances/UCM193282.pdf

54. Kawata AK, Hsieh R, Bender R, Shaffer S, Revicki DA, Bayliss M, et al. Psychometric evaluation of a novel instrument assessing the impact of migraine on physical functioning: the migraine physical function impact diary. Headache. 2017;57:1385–98.

55. Hareendran A, Skalicky A, Mannix S, Lavoie S, Desai P, Bayliss M, et al. Development of a new tool for evaluating the benefit of preventive treatments for migraine on functional outcomes – the Migraine Functional Impact Questionnaire (MFIQ). Headache. 2018;58(10):1612–28.

56. Kawata AK, Hareendran A, Shaffer S, Mannix S, Thach A, Desai P, et al. Evaluating the psychometric properties of the Migraine Functional Impact Questionnaire (MFIQ). Headache. 2019;59(8):1253–69.

57. Lerner D, Amick BC III, Malspeis S, Rogers WH, Santanello N, Gerth W, et al. The migraine work and productivity loss questionnaire: concepts and design. Qual Life Res. 1999;8:699–710.

58. Davies GM, Santanello N, Gerth W, Lerner D, Block GA. Validation of a migraine work and productivity loss questionnaire for use in migraine studies. Cephalalgia. 1999;19:497–502.

59. Mushet GR, Miller D, Clements B, Pait DG, Gutterman D. Impact of sumatriptan on workplace productivity, nonwork activities, and health-related quality of life among hospital employees with migraine. Headache. 1996:137–43.
60. D'Amico D, Grazzi L, Grignani E, Leonardi M, Sansone E, Raggi A, HEADWORK Study Group. HEADWORK questionnaire: why do we need a new tool to assess work-related disability in patients with migraine? Headache. 2020;60(2):497–504.
61. Raggi A, Covelli V, Guastafierro E, Leonardi M, Scaratti C, Grazzi L, et al. Validation of a self-reported instrument to assess work-related difficulties in patients with migraine: the HEADWORK questionnaire. J Headache Pain. 2018;19(1):85.

# Chapter 8
# Patient-Reported Outcomes in Migraine and Cluster Headache

Helin Gosalia, David Moreno-Ajona, and Peter J. Goadsby

## 8.1 Introduction

The importance of primary headache disorders has been under-appreciated by the medical community for many years. Awareness of its impact on the patient population has increased its relevance, although not to a degree that matches its place in causes of global disability [1]. Given the disabling nature of primary headache disorders, patient-reported outcomes (PROs) are crucial to understand better the efficacy of treatments, address the severity of the disorder and understand disease progression. The United States Food and Drug Administration defines patient-reported outcome (PRO) as a measurement established from a report given by the patient directly about the status of a patient's health condition without modification or interpretation of the patient's response by a clinician or anyone else [2]. Medical technology provides biochemical or physiological data, however, data concerning treatment, disease pathology or quality of life can only be captured from the patient directly. Considering that migraine and cluster headache, specifically, have no current curative treatment, obtaining PROs are important for evaluating treatment pathways. Generic health-related quality of life scales have also been used in the field. Stafford and colleagues conducted a study administering the EQ-5D™ to 106 migraineurs to assess the varying levels of migraine pain severity on utility values

H. Gosalia · D. Moreno-Ajona
NIHR SLaM Clinical Research Facility, King's College London, London, UK

P. J. Goadsby (✉)
NIHR SLaM Clinical Research Facility, King's College London, London, UK

King's College Hospital, London, UK
e-mail: peter.goadsby@kcl.ac.uk



P. Yalınay Dikmen, A. Özge (eds.), *Clinical Scales for Headache Disorders*, Headache, https://doi.org/10.1007/978-3-031-25938-8_8

**Table 8.1** Generic headache patient-reported outcome measures

| Patient-report outcome measure | Acronym | Measure overview |
| --- | --- | --- |
| Headache Impact Test [7, 8] | HIT | A broad measure for patients to relay the impact of their headaches |
| Headache Impact Test-6 [9] | HIT-6 | A six-item short-form measure for patients to relay the impact of their headaches |
| Headache Disability Questionnaire [10] | HDQ | A headache-specific disability measure for patients receiving physiotherapy treatment for their headaches |
| EUROLIGHT Questionnaire [11] | – | A measure used to assess and evaluate the burden of primary headache disorders |
| Headache Activities of Daily Living Index [12] | HADLI | A measure used to assess headache-related disability concentrating on important activities of daily living |

and health statuses. The authors concluded that higher levels of migraine pain resulted in lower levels of utility. Nonetheless, experiencing a migraine, irrespective of pain intensity, led to reduced utility overall [3]. There are five generic headache PRO measures that have been developed, with a particular focus on quality of life (see Table 8.1). On the other hand, Patient Global Impression of Change (PGIC) [4] is a very practical tool [5] which is commonly used in clinical trials [6].

The most commonly used of them all are the Headache Impact Test (HIT) [7, 8] and the Headache Impact Test-6 [9]. Primary headache research has utilised these measures to aid our understanding and they have been useful and reliable tools [13, 14].

## 8.2 PROs in Migraine

Headache disorders are the second leading cause of disability-adjusted life-years in ages 10–24 years and the fifth for 25–49 years [1]. Migraine, specifically, is a severely disabling brain disorder. Understanding the impact of the disorder on patients' quality of life, well-being and treatment efficacy allows clinicians to understand further the disorder and in turn, address areas of concern (Table 8.2).

Many PRO instruments have been used in recent years to obtain data in migraine. Examples of such instruments are; the Migraine Disability Assessment (MIDAS) [17, 18], the Migraine-Specific Quality of Life Questionnaire (MSQOL) [15, 16] and the Migraine-Specific Quality of Life Questionnaire version 2.1 (MSQ v2.1) [19]. These validated assessments quantify headache-related disability and evaluate the impact headache has on aspects of social life, professional life and communicate how patients feel as a result of the headache-related impact. Whilst such validated measures have been important to our understanding of the magnitude to which migraine affects the patient population, it is essential to understand the effect migraine has on patients. This can facilitate treatment pathways and enrich our understanding of migraine pathophysiology. PRO instruments such as the Migraine

**Table 8.2**  Migraine-specific patient-reported outcome measures

| Patient-report outcome measure | Acronym | Measure overview |
|---|---|---|
| Migraine-Specific Quality of Life Questionnaire [15, 16] | MSQOL | A measure used to assess quality of life for migraine patients, covering three domains; avoidance behaviours, social relations and feelings |
| Migraine Disability Assessment [17, 18] | MIDAS | A measure used to quantify headache-related disability, with a broad reference to 'headache' |
| Migraine-Specific Quality of Life Questionnaire version 2.1 [19] | MSQ v2.1 | A measure used to assess quality of life for migraine patients, covering three domains; role restrictive, role preventive and emotional functioning |
| Headache Needs Assessment [20] | HANA | A migraine-specific health-related quality of life measure, particularly assessing 'frequency' and 'bothersomeness' |
| Migraine Therapy Assessment Questionnaire [21] | M-TAQ | A measure used to assess patients whose migraine management may be suboptimal in a primary care setting |
| Migraine Treatment Satisfaction Measure [22] | MTSM | A measure used to evaluate satisfaction with migraine treatment |
| Migraine Assessment of Current Therapy [23] | Migraine-ACT | A measure used to identify patients who need a change in their current acute migraine treatment |
| Functional Assessment in Migraine [24] | FAIM | A measure used to assess functional status associated with migraine |
| Patient Perception of Migraine Questionnaire-Revised [25] | PPMQ-R | A revised measure to assess patient satisfaction with acute migraine therapy |
| Migraine-Treatment Optimization Questionnaire [26] | M-TOQ | A measure used to assess response to acute migraine treatment in migraineurs |
| Completeness of Response Survey [27] | CORS | A measure used to assess factors important to patients when considering the commencement and continuation of migraine treatment |
| Activity Impairment in Migraine Diary [28] | AIM-D | A psychometrically sound measure to assess the functional impact of migraine |

Treatment Satisfaction (MTSM) [22] and the Patient Perception of Migraine Questionnaire-Revised (PPMQ-R) [25] are aimed to assess migraine treatment and satisfaction. These measures aid understanding of current migraine treatment and help evaluate novel therapies.

## 8.2.1  Premonitory Symptoms

As migraine is better understood, PROs need to evolve. In recent years attention has been drawn to the premonitory stage and its symptoms [29]. The presence of these non-headache symptoms, typically present before the onset of an attack, occurring from hours to up to a day or two before the onset of attack symptomology, is defined as the premonitory phase [29, 30]. To date, PROs have been focused on measuring pain, with a few questionnaires addressing cognitive symptoms [31]. In our clinic we ask patients about the presence of premonitory symptoms, such as mood changes, irritability, lethargy, yawning, neck stiffness, cognitive impairment or brain fog, difficulty concentrating, food craving, food aversion, changes to bowel or bladder habits, routinely to phenotype patients thoroughly and build an understanding of the neurobiology [32]. Obtaining this information creates a dataset that can be used to increase understanding and recognition of the premonitory phase by patients and physicians [30]. Furthermore, awareness of these symptoms may warn patients of an attack. Neuroimaging studies have demonstrated a focal role of the hypothalamus, midbrain and the limbic pathways potentially involved in the premonitory phase [33]. Initial studies investigating the premonitory phase of migraine using blood flow as a surrogate of neuronal activation recognised areas, such as the hypothalamus [33]. Furthermore, more novel measurement techniques assessing blood flow changes through the course of the premonitory phase correlated with the earlier findings [34]. A wider recognition by patients of premonitory symptoms may facilitate research on essentially manipulating the biology during the infancy of an attack and open treatment pathways that avert migraine attacks.

### 8.2.2 Migraine Triggers

Another notable feature of migraine pathophysiology are the so-called triggers. Many migraineurs will report triggers or factors that are likely to increase the possibility of an attack [32, 35]. However, it is interesting to note that there may be some subtle differences between premonitory symptoms and triggers, which are not so distinct for both patients and clinicians. For example, chocolate or sugary food was thought to be a trigger and more so now the craving for sugar is thought to be a premonitory symptom. In theory, an understanding of migraine triggers may essentially prevent the onset of an attack, by taking preventive therapeutics and further allowing patients a sense of management over the disorder. In our clinic, we address migraine triggers by asking patients about the following: alcohol (within minutes or the next day), menstrual cycle, stress, relaxation from stress, oversleeping, undersleeping, skipping meals, dehydration, hot weather, stormy weather, etc. [35]. We also ask about position and Valsalva manoeuvres, such as coughing, bowel movements, bending and physical exertion, to exclude 'red flags.' These are symptoms of concern or true 'red flags,' they are actual triggers, not worsening factors, to distinguish this is important. To date, there is no PRO instrument addressing the premonitory features of migraine; such a development would improve our understanding of the disorder and its management. Moreover, PRO instruments could aid clinical trials to understand new approaches to treatment.

## 8.3 PROs in Cluster Headache

In a recent report, cluster headache patients described the attacks as the most painful affliction experienced [36]. The intensity and severity of the pain has given the disorder the epithet 'suicide headache.' A better understanding of the effect on patients' daily lives, treatment efficacy, quality of life and associated symptoms, will allow the medical community to understand better the disorder and thus help patients. It is interesting to note that in migraine attacks the associated cranial autonomic symptoms tend to be less severe [37], given the higher prevalence of migraine, more literature has been devoted to migraine PROs compared to cluster headache. The biology, presentation of symptoms, classification and even types of attacks differ between these two primary headache disorders and thus, specificity in terms of measuring PROs is imperative. As highlighted above, there is a portfolio of PRO measures particularly investigating quality of life in migraine. However, there is a paucity of measures investigating this in cluster headache. Moreover, studies have utilised migraine-specific measures or generic quality of life measures [38, 39] to assess quality of life in cluster headache patients as they have a common dominant symptom, headache. Ertsey and colleagues [38] adopted the MSQ v2.1 [19] to examine and evaluate health-related quality of life in patients presenting with episodic cluster headache [38]. Their findings highlighted that the cluster headache patients had lower scores for all tested measures, showing impaired health-related quality of life [38]. It is noteworthy that there was a statistically significant difference in health-related quality of life between cluster headache patients but not between cluster headache patients and migraine patients [38]. Given the obvious differences in pain intensity, longevity and disorder biology, the use of a migraine-specific measure is questioned. These scales may not be able to quantify the true effects of cluster headache and consequently, misinterpreting the impact of the disorder on the patient population. In more recent years, cluster headache-specific measures have been developed (see Table 8.3).

Abu Bakar and colleagues developed and validated the first PRO instrument to measure quality of life in cluster headache sufferers [40]. This measure was developed specifically for the disorder. The development of the scale has been a useful advance in understanding the specific quality of life impairment, disorder associated difficulties and for use as a PRO assessment in research and a clinical setting.

**Table 8.3** Cluster headache-specific patient-reported outcome measures

| Patient-report outcome measure | Acronym | Measure overview |
| --- | --- | --- |
| Cluster Headache Quality of Life Scale [40] | CHQ | A cluster headache-specific quality of life scale |
| Cluster Headache Scales [41] | CHS | A broad-spectrum measure of psychosocial factors in cluster headache |
| Cluster Headache Impact Questionnaire [42] | CHIQ | A cluster headache-specific disability measure, assessing the impact of cluster headache on daily life |

Additionally, the Cluster Headache Scales (CHS) have been developed to assess psychosocial factors in cluster headache [41]. More recently, a cluster headache-related disability assessment has been developed, the Cluster Headache Impact Questionnaire (CHIQ) [42]. This addresses more disorder-specific questions such as the unpredictability of attacks and self-injurious behaviour due to attack pain intensity [42]. Taking patients into consideration is very important when developing PROs, given they are able to provide the best insight, it is useful to take their experience onboard as it will enable physicians to better meet patient needs. The Kip Scale, was devised by a long-term cluster headache sufferer, as a means to standardise cluster headache sufferers' pain description [43]. This scale is of valuable use to patients when describing their pain in a clinical setting. Moving forward, physicians and researchers would benefit from the patient populations input when developing novel PRO scales.

On the contrary, in tandem with migraine PROs, there is a general lack of instruments covering biology-specific questions which assess beyond quality of life measures. Quality of life evaluation is key, but we cannot improve patient quality of life unless we better understand disorder-specific characteristics. Employing novel instruments to assess PROs in cluster headache will stimulate and channel research for efficacious treatments that prevent the disabling effects of the disorder. Moreover, considering the nature of cluster headache and the bouts, if a generic headache or migraine-specific questionnaire is administered, for example, the patient may have been out of their bout, for some time before the questionnaire administration. In which case, the data captured would not reflect the true effects of the disorder. Furthermore, periodicity is unique to cluster headache biology [44]. The pain associated tends to be usually around the same time, this periodicity is typical for cluster headache and not for other primary headache disorders [45, 46]. Therefore, this further stipulates the necessity for more cluster headache-specific PRO instruments. Additionally, cluster headache is often associated with consequential psychiatric tendencies [46], such as depression and anxiety [47, 48]. The disabling nature of the disorder warrants early diagnosis and interventions to manage the pain. To assess the magnitude to which this affects sufferers, primary reports via PROs are essential.

Aside from symptomology, cluster headache treatment requires an assessment of current treatment options and newly emerging treatment pathways. For example, a treatment that is unique to cluster headache is the inhalation of 100% high flow oxygen [49]. This treatment is distinctive to this primary headache disorder alone. High flow oxygen treatment for 15 minutes is currently the safest and most effective acute treatment [49, 50]. However, around 20% of patients do not benefit from this treatment [50] and it is yet to be elucidated how this treatment is efficacious for those with cluster headache. Naturally, the patient population is able to provide a better insight into treatment efficacy. Apropos treatment, it is vital we ask patients questions about their treatment plans (both acute and preventive), with specific details such as dosage. Therefore, noting a patient as a non-responder to a particular drug, without specific details, which in a clinical trial for example, may bias the data. Without the specific dosage details, one cannot say if they are non-responders as they did not take it at the relevant dose or the relevant duration. This highlights the importance of PROs also in a research setting as well as a clinical setting. Without targeted, disorder-specific PRO instruments, we cannot understand if the treatment options are successful and how we may better the treatment pathways. One may argue that administering PRO instruments that are not disorder-specific may actually be counterproductive and create datasets that are misleading and not a true representative of the disorder, as each disorder has unique presentations. It is noteworthy that one of the most disabling disorders known to mankind has not motivated adequate research around PROs in cluster headache. There is an urgent necessity to collect PRO data on cluster headache, allowing clinicians and researchers to steer research in a patient-oriented direction.

## 8.4 Conclusion

Ultimately, the medical and scientific community seeks to improve the lives of those suffering from primary headache disorders. By considering primary source data via PROs, there is a substantial opportunity to evolve the field. In order to better the lives of those suffering from disorders such as cluster headache and migraine, we must capture their assessment of treatment options, quality of life and symptomatology. To date, we have some useful tools and we have been addressing the disability, impact on lives and efficacy of new treatments and there is room for improvement in the field.

## References


1. Diseases GBD, Injuries C. Global burden of 369 diseases and injuries in 204 countries and territories, 1990-2019: a systematic analysis for the Global Burden of Disease Study 2019. Lancet. 2020;396(10258):1204–22. https://doi.org/10.1016/S0140-6736(20)30925-9.
2. U.S. Department of Health and Human Services FDA Center for Drug Evaluation and Research, U.S. Department of Health and Human Services FDA Center for Biologics Evaluation and Research & U.S. Department of Health and Human Services FDA Center for Devices and Radiological Health. Guidance for industry: patient-reported outcome measures: use in medical product development to support labeling claims: draft guidance. Health Qual Life Outcomes. 2006;4:79. https://doi.org/10.1186/1477-7525-4-79.
3. Stafford MR, Hareendran A, Ng-Mak DS, Insinga RP, Xu R, Stull DE. EQ-5D-derived utility values for different levels of migraine severity from a UK sample of migraineurs. Health Qual Life Outcomes. 2012;10:65. https://doi.org/10.1186/1477-7525-10-65.
4. Hurst H, Bolton J. Assessing the clinical significance of change scores recorded on subjective outcome measures. J Manipulative Physiol Ther. 2004;27(1):26–35. https://doi.org/10.1016/j.jmpt.2003.11.003.
5. Alpuente A, Gallardo VJ, Caronna E, Torres-Ferrus M, Pozo-Rosich P. In search of a gold standard patient-reported outcome measure to use in the evaluation and treatment-decision making in migraine prevention. A real-world evidence study. J Headache Pain. 2021;22(1):151. https://doi.org/10.1186/s10194-021-01366-9.

6. McGinley JS, Houts CR, Nishida TK, Buse DC, Lipton RB, Goadsby PJ, et al. Systematic review of outcomes and endpoints in preventive migraine clinical trials. Headache. 2021;61(2):253–62. https://doi.org/10.1111/head.14069.

7. Bjorner JB, Kosinski M, Ware JE Jr. Calibration of an item pool for assessing the burden of headaches: an application of item response theory to the headache impact test (HIT). Qual Life Res. 2003;12(8):913–33. https://doi.org/10.1023/A:1026163113446.

8. Ware JE Jr, Kosinski M, Bjorner JB, Bayliss MS, Batenhorst A, Dahlof CG, et al. Applications of computerized adaptive testing (CAT) to the assessment of headache impact. Qual Life Res. 2003;12(8):935–52. https://doi.org/10.1023/A:1026115230284.

9. Kosinski M, Bayliss MS, Bjorner JB, Ware JE Jr, Garber WH, Batenhorst A, et al. A six-item short-form survey for measuring headache impact: the HIT-6. Qual Life Res. 2003;12(8):963–74. https://doi.org/10.1023/A:1026119331193.

10. Niere K, Quin A. Development of a headache-specific disability questionnaire for patients attending physiotherapy. Man Ther. 2009;14(1):45–51. https://doi.org/10.1016/j.math.2007.09.006.

11. Andree C, Vaillant M, Barre J, Katsarava Z, Lainez JM, Lair ML, et al. Development and validation of the EUROLIGHT questionnaire to evaluate the burden of primary headache disorders in Europe. Cephalalgia. 2010;30(9):1082–100. https://doi.org/10.1177/2F0333102409354323.

12. Vernon H, Lawson G. Development of the headache activities of daily living index: initial validity study. J Manipulative Physiol Ther. 2015;38(2):102–11. https://doi.org/10.1016/j.jmpt.2014.12.002.

13. Houts CR, McGinley JS, Wirth RJ, Cady R, Lipton RB. Reliability and validity of the 6-item Headache Impact Test in chronic migraine from the PROMISE-2 study. Qual Life Res. 2021;30(3):931–43. https://doi.org/10.1007/s11136-020-02668-2.

14. Barloese MC, Jurgens TP, May A, Lainez JM, Schoenen J, Gaul C, et al. Cluster headache attack remission with sphenopalatine ganglion stimulation: experiences in chronic cluster headache patients through 24 months. J Headache Pain. 2016;17(1):67. https://doi.org/10.1186/s10194-016-0658-1.

15. McKenna SP, Doward LC, Davey KM. The development and psychometric properties of the MSQOL: a migraine-specific quality-of-life instrument. Clin Drug Investig. 1998;15(5):413–23. https://doi.org/10.2165/00044011-199815050-00006.

16. Wagner TH, Patrick DL, Galer BS, Berzon RA. A new instrument to assess the long-term quality of life effects from migraine: development and psychometric testing of the MSQOL. Headache. 1996;36(8):484–92. https://doi.org/10.1046/j.1526-4610.1996.3608484.x.

17. Stewart WF, Lipton RB, Kolodner K, Liberman J, Sawyer J. Reliability of the migraine disability assessment score in a population-based sample of headache sufferers. Cephalalgia. 1999;19(2):107–14.; Discussion 74. https://doi.org/10.1046/j.1468-2982.1999.019002107.x.

18. Stewart WF, Lipton RB, Dowson AJ, Sawyer J. Development and testing of the Migraine Disability Assessment (MIDAS) Questionnaire to assess headache-related disability. Neurology. 2001;56(6 Suppl 1):S20–8. https://doi.org/10.1212/WNL.56.suppl_1.S20.

19. Martin BC, Pathak DS, Sharfman MI, Adelman JU, Taylor F, Kwong WJ, et al. Validity and reliability of the migraine-specific quality of life questionnaire (MSQ Version 2.1). Headache. 2000;40(3):204–15. https://doi.org/10.1046/j.1526-4610.2000.00030.x.

20. Cramer JA, Silberstein SD, Winner P. Development and validation of the Headache Needs Assessment (HANA) survey. Headache. 2001;41(4):402–9. https://doi.org/10.1046/j.1526-4610.2001.111006402.x.

21. Chatterton ML, Lofland JH, Shechter A, Curtice WS, Hu XH, Lenow J, et al. Reliability and validity of the migraine therapy assessment questionnaire. Headache. 2002;42(10):1006–15. https://doi.org/10.1046/j.1526-4610.2002.02230.x.

22. Patrick DL, Martin ML, Bushnell DM, Pesa J. Measuring satisfaction with migraine treatment: expectations, importance, outcomes, and global ratings. Clin Ther. 2003;25(11):2920–35. https://doi.org/10.1016/S0149-2918(03)80345-4.

23. Dowson AJ, D'Amico D, Tepper SJ, Baos V, Baudet F, Kilminster S. Identifying patients who require a change in their current acute migraine treatment: the Migraine Assessment of Current Therapy (Migraine-ACT) questionnaire. Neurol Sci. 2004;25(Suppl 3):S276–8. https://doi.org/10.1007/s10072-004-0308-2.
24. Pathak DS, Chisolm DJ, Weis KA. Functional Assessment in Migraine (FAIM) questionnaire: development of an instrument based upon the WHO's International Classification of Functioning, Disability, and Health. Value Health. 2005;8(5):591–600. https://doi.org/10.1111/j.1524-4733.2005.00047.x.
25. Kimel M, Hsieh R, McCormack J, Burch SP, Revicki DA. Validation of the revised Patient Perception of Migraine Questionnaire (PPMQ-R): measuring satisfaction with acute migraine treatment in clinical trials. Cephalalgia. 2008;28(5):510–23. https://doi.org/10.1111/j.1468-2982.2007.01524.x.
26. Lipton RB, Kolodner K, Bigal ME, Valade D, Lainez MJ, Pascual J, et al. Validity and reliability of the Migraine-Treatment Optimization Questionnaire. Cephalalgia. 2009;29(7):751–9. https://doi.org/10.1111/j.1468-2982.2008.01786.x.
27. Coon CD, Fehnel SE, Davis KH, Runken MC, Beach ME, Cady RK. The development of a survey to measure completeness of response to migraine therapy. Headache. 2012;52(4):550–72. https://doi.org/10.1111/j.1526-4610.2012.02099.x.
28. Lipton RB, Gandhi P, Stokes J, Cala ML, Evans CJ, Knoble N, et al. Development and validation of a novel patient-reported outcome measure in people with episodic migraine and chronic migraine: The Activity Impairment in Migraine Diary. Headache. 2022;62(1):89–105. https://doi.org/10.1111/head.14229.
29. Giffin NJ, Ruggiero L, Lipton RB, Silberstein SD, Tvedskov JF, Olesen J, et al. Premonitory symptoms in migraine: an electronic diary study. Neurology. 2003;60(6):935–40. https://doi.org/10.1212/01.WNL.0000052998.58526.A9.
30. Karsan N, Goadsby PJ. Biological insights from the premonitory symptoms of migraine. Nat Rev Neurol. 2018;14(12):699–710. https://doi.org/10.1038/s41582-018-0098-4.
31. Gil-Gouveia R, Oliveira AG, Martins IP. A subjective cognitive impairment scale for migraine attacks. The MIG-SCOG: development and validation. Cephalalgia. 2011;31(9):984–91. https://doi.org/10.1177/0333102411408359.
32. Goadsby PJ, Holland PR, Martins-Oliveira M, Hoffmann J, Schankin C, Akerman S. Pathophysiology of migraine: a disorder of sensory processing. Physiol Rev. 2017;97(2):553–622. https://doi.org/10.1152/physrev.00034.2015.
33. Maniyar FH, Sprenger T, Monteith T, Schankin C, Goadsby PJ. Brain activations in the premonitory phase of nitroglycerin-triggered migraine attacks. Brain. 2014;137(Pt 1):232–41. https://doi.org/10.1093/brain/awt320.
34. Karsan N, Bose P, Zelaya FO, Goadsby PJ. Alterations in cerebral blood flow associated with the premonitory phase of migraine. Cephalalgia. 2018;38:36.
35. Karsan N, Bose P, Newman J, Goadsby PJ. Are some patient-perceived migraine triggers simply early manifestations of the attack? J Neurol. 2021;268(5):1885–93. https://doi.org/10.1007/s00415-020-10344-1.
36. Burish MJ, Pearson SM, Shapiro RE, Zhang W, Schor LI. Cluster headache is one of the most intensely painful human conditions: Results from the International Cluster Headache Questionnaire. Headache. 2021;61(1):117–24. https://doi.org/10.1111/head.14021.
37. Lai TH, Fuh JL, Wang SJ. Cranial autonomic symptoms in migraine: characteristics and comparison with cluster headache. J Neurol Neurosurg Psychiatry. 2009;80(10):1116–9. https://doi.org/10.1136/jnnp.2008.157743.
38. Ertsey C, Manhalter N, Bozsik G, Afra J, Jelencsik I. Health-related and condition-specific quality of life in episodic cluster headache. Cephalalgia. 2004;24(3):188–96. https://doi.org/10.1111/j.1468-2982.2003.00655.x.
39. D'Amico D, Rigamonti A, Solari A, Leone M, Usai S, Grazzi L, et al. Health-related quality of life in patients with cluster headache during active periods. Cephalalgia. 2002;22(10):818–21. https://doi.org/10.1046/j.1468-2982.2002.00463.x.

40. Abu Bakar N, Torkamani M, Tanprawate S, Lambru G, Matharu M, Jahanshahi M. The development and validation of the Cluster Headache Quality of life scale (CHQ). J Headache Pain. 2016;17(1):79. https://doi.org/10.1186/s10194-016-0674-1.

41. Klan T, Brascher AK, Vales A, Liesering-Latta E, Witthoft M, Gaul C. Determination of psychosocial factors in cluster headache—construction and psychometric properties of the Cluster Headache Scales (CHS). Cephalalgia. 2020;40(11):1240–9. https://doi.org/10.1177/0333102420928076.

42. Kamm K, Straube A, Ruscheweyh R. Cluster Headache Impact Questionnaire (CHIQ)—a short measure of cluster headache related disability. J Headache Pain. 2022;23(1):37. https://doi.org/10.1186/s10194-022-01406-y.

43. Kipple B. The Kip Scale: Organisation for understanding cluster headache—UK; 2014. Available from http://ouchuk.org/sites/default/files/downloads/kip_scale_0.pdf.

44. Kunkle EC, Pfeiffer JB, Jr., Wilhoit WM, Hamrick LW, Jr. Recurrent brief headache in cluster pattern. Trans Am Neurol Assoc. 1952;56(77th Meeting):240–3.

45. Dodick DW, Capobianco DJ. Treatment and management of cluster headache. Curr Pain Headache Rep. 2001;5(1):83–91. https://doi.org/10.1007/s11916-001-0015-0.

46. Hoffmann J, May A. Diagnosis, pathophysiology, and management of cluster headache. Lancet Neurol. 2018;17(1):75–83. https://doi.org/10.1016/S1474-4422(17)30405-2.

47. Louter MA, Wilbrink LA, Haan J, van Zwet EW, van Oosterhout WP, Zitman FG, et al. Cluster headache and depression. Neurology. 2016;87(18):1899–906. https://doi.org/10.1212/WNL.0000000000003282.

48. Jorge RE, Leston JE, Arndt S, Robinson RG. Cluster headaches: association with anxiety disorders and memory deficits. Neurology. 1999;53(3):543–7. https://doi.org/10.1212/WNL.53.3.543.

49. Cohen AS, Burns B, Goadsby PJ. High-flow oxygen for treatment of cluster headache: a randomized trial. JAMA. 2009;302(22):2451–7. https://doi.org/10.1001/jama.2009.1855.

50. Fogan L. Treatment of cluster headache. A double-blind comparison of oxygen v air inhalation. Arch Neurol. 1985;42(4):362–3. https://doi.org/10.1001/archneur.1985.04060040072015.

# Chapter 9
# Clinical Scales for Psychiatric Comorbidities and Cognitive Processes in Headache and Migraine

Valeria Caponnetto, Chiara Rosignoli, and Simona Sacco

## 9.1 Introduction

Primary headache disorders are considered neurological chronic disorders with episodic manifestations (CDEM) featured with recurrent attacks and return to baseline during interictal stages. The co-existence of these disorders with psychiatric disorders might be expected due to a possible bidirectional relationship that includes mutual causality, latent brain state models, shared precipitating environment, and shared genetic origins [1–3]. The epidemiology of this co-existence has been more deeply investigated regarding migraine rather than cluster headache or tension type headache [2]. However, it seems that psychiatric disorders are among the most common comorbidities in primary headache patients [2] and their prevalence seems to be higher in these patients when compared to general population [4, 5].

In particular, migraineurs often present other neurological or psychiatric comorbidities, including mood disorders. In this regard, migraine requires special attention since migraine patients reported a higher probability to have psychiatric comorbidities, such as major depression, anxiety, panic disorder, posttraumatic stress disorder (PTSD), or suicidal behavior, with higher rates in chronic migraine compared to episodic migraine [3, 6].

In addition to psychiatric comorbidities, patients with headaches have an increased risk of developing cognitive impairment or enacting dysfunctional cognitive styles that can lead to chronification of attacks. Headache patients, and

V. Caponnetto · C. Rosignoli · S. Sacco (✉)
Department of Biotechnological and Applied Clinical Sciences, University of L'Aquila, Coppito, L'Aquila, Italy
e-mail: valeria.caponnetto@univaq.it; chiara.rosignoli@graduate.univaq.it; simona.sacco@univaq.it



P. Yalınay Dikmen, A. Özge (eds.), *Clinical Scales for Headache Disorders*, Headache, https://doi.org/10.1007/978-3-031-25938-8_9

specifically migraineurs, show cognitive impairment during attacks. The cognitive domains that appear to be most dysfunctional are processing speed, memory, executive functions and verbal skills [7].

Cognitive styles, on the other hand, influence the behavior of patients not only during the migraine attack. They refer to the beliefs, perceptions, and thinking styles inherent to pathology and pain perception. People with headache differ to healthy control in emotional distress, locus of control, coping strategies, illness perceptions and pain catastrophizing [8, 9].

A proper assessment of psychiatric comorbidities and cognitive processes is fundamental in order to properly understand patients' features and needs and orient therapeutic strategies [6].

## 9.2 Clinical Scales for Psychiatric Comorbidities in Headache and Migraine

Many clinical instruments may be used in clinical practice and studies to suggest a diagnosis of psychiatric disorders or detect psychiatric symptoms in migraine patients. In fact, some instruments are considered as screening, while others only allow to detect symptoms related to psychiatric disorders.

When choosing an instrument for clinical practice or research, some preliminary considerations should be performed by answering the following questions:

- Does the feature assessed through the instrument fit with clinical/research aims?
- Is the instrument developed for your target population and setting?
- Is the instrument available in the desired language and which are its use terms & conditions?
- If the instrument allows to detect psychiatric symptoms, is it valid and reliable (see Chap. 3)?
- If the instrument allows to suggest a diagnosis of psychiatric disorders (screening), what is its sensitivity and specificity towards the gold standard?
- For research projects: was the instrument used in similar studies to allow literature outcomes' comparisons? [10]

Considering most common psychiatric disorders in migraineurs, we describe widely used instruments to suggest their diagnosis or evaluate the presence of their symptoms.

### 9.2.1 *Personality Traits and Mood or Anxiety Disorder*

**1. Minnesota Multiphasic Personality Inventory (MMPI)**
The original MMPI was published in 1942 to assess psychiatric problems in different settings, and it is currently widely used. It was revised in 1989, leading to an

adult (MMPI-2) and adolescent (MMPI-A) version. Through 478 items, MMPI-2 allows to delineate a general personality profile and clinical symptoms, assessing subjects' symptoms, beliefs, and attitudes. However, empirical research conducted by original authors allowed to identify groups of items able to discriminate subjects with possible psychiatric conditions, such as hypochondriasis, depression, hysteria, psychopathic deviation, paranoid thinking, psychasthenia, schizophrenia, mania, sex role identification, and social introversion and extraversion. However, a plethora of scales grouping different items of MMPI-2 have been developed so far and their rationale and validity are not always clear [11].

Items are answered through a true-false scale and total scoring is conducted through a normalization algorithm calculating a possible score ranging from 30 to 120 with scores above 65 considered as clinically significant. Moreover, when scoring, not only single scales can be considered, but also patterns of multiple scales [11, 12].

This scale has been widely used in chronic pain and headache, producing controversial results among different primary headache disorders [13, 14].

## 2. My Mood Monitor (M-3) Checklist

This scale was validated in English in 2010 as a screening tool against the historical instrument Mini International Neuropsychiatric Interview (MINI) [15]. M-3 checklist evaluates the presence of depressive, bipolar, anxiety, and PTSD through 27 patient-rated items with a 5-level Likert scale from 0 ('not at all') to 4 ('most of the time'). Patients are asked to indicate whether and how often they experienced, during the past 2 weeks, symptoms of major depressive disorder (seven questions, including a suicide question), generalized anxiety disorder (two questions), panic disorder (two questions), social anxiety disorder (one question), post-traumatic stress disorder (four questions), and obsessive-compulsive disorder (three questions), lifetime history of symptoms of the bipolar spectrum disorder (four questions), and functional impairment (four questions) [16].

For scoring, first of all, the suicide and functional impairment questions have to be considered. If these are answered 'not at all', patient score is zero and they are considered not suitable for psychiatric disorder diagnosis. If one or more of these questions was answered differently from 'not at all', sub-scores of the other four diagnostic categories should summed considering the following coding protocol: 'not at all' and 'rarely' = 0, 'sometimes' = 1, and 'often' and 'most of the time' = 2. Hence, final possible score ranges between 0 and 44, with higher scores indicating higher possibility to diagnose mood disorders [16].

Reported sensitivity was 0.83 and specificity 0.76 for any mood or anxiety disorder. Moreover, sensitivity and specificity for each disorder allowed to consider this instrument as accurate as instruments that detect single disorders. Therefore, disorder-specific items could be utilized if needed [16].

It requires less than 5 min for the patient to fill the questionnaire and its scoring is quick, though quite complex; the ideal setting of use is primary care [16].

Although its use is mainly suggested in primary care, it might be suggested also in headache patients considering quick of use and accurateness. Moreover, this would allow to compare headache patients with other populations through research results.

## *9.2.2 Anxiety and Depression*

Symptoms related to these disorders are among the most investigated in headache patients and the following described scales are often included in epidemiological studies and studies evaluating treatments results [17–22].

### 9.2.2.1 Anxiety

**1. Generalized Anxiety Disorder-7 (GAD-7)**

GAD-7 was validated in English 2006 as an instrument suggesting the presence of symptoms related to generalized anxiety disorder in the last 2 weeks. Patients are asked to indicate how often they were bothered by each symptom (7 items) through a 7-items and 4-level Likert scale from 0 ('not at all') to 3 ('nearly every day') [23].

For scoring, items scores are summed with a total possible score ranging between 0 and 21 and higher scores indicating higher presence of GAD symptoms. Proposed cut-off for interpretation were 5, 10, and 15, that correspond to probable mild, moderate, and severe levels of anxiety [23].

Its divergent validity was assessed towards the 8-item Patient Health Questionnaire (PHQ-8) depression score, while convergent validity was assessed towards Beck Anxiety Inventory (BAI), and the anxiety subscale of the Symptom Checklist-90, since there were no other scales specific for GAD. Moreover, its construct validity was assessed towards Short-Form General Health Survey (SF-20) functional status scales, self-reported disability days, and physician visits. These analyses and results from other studies showed good psychometric properties of the GAD-7 in primary care and general population, since this scale revealed able to identify probable cases of GAD, discriminate its severity, and clearly identify anxiety rather than depression symptoms [23]. Also brief versions of the scale showed similar results, i.e. GAD-2 and GAD-Single Item (GAD-SI). These scales include two and one GAD-7 core questions, respectively, and showed a similar ability to detect GAD symptoms. Answers and scoring algorithm are the same as GAD-7. Moreover, all the described versions could be useful and reliable tools to screen for panic disorder, social phobia, and PTSD [24].

This scale offers the possibility to quickly and easily assess the presence of anxiety symptoms in the last 2 weeks, though it is not clear if it is able to detect long-term changes [23].

**2. Beck Anxiety Inventory (BAI)**

This scale was developed in English in 1988, and revised in 1993 regarding scoring, to assess anxiety severity, mainly in psychiatric patients. It is a patient-rated 21-items scale with a 4-levels Likert-scale ranging from 0 ('not at all') to 3 ('severely'). Patients are asked to indicate how much they have been bothered by described anxiety symptoms in the last week [25, 26].

Items scores are summed to obtain a total score ranging from 0 to 63 with higher scores indicating more severe anxiety symptoms. Patients can be classified as presenting minimal, mild, moderate, and severe anxiety considering score ranges of 0–7, 8–15, 15–25, and above 25, respectively [25, 26].

Though showing to be able to discriminate well between anxious and nonanxious patients with good reliability, the literature also showed high correlation of BAI with Beck Depression Inventory-II (BDI-II) [27], suggesting to considering the diagnostic ability of this scale with caution. However, it requires few minutes to be filled and its scoring is quick, leading to consider it as a possible screening tool and support for diagnosis [25, 26].

### 9.2.2.2  Depression

**1. Beck Depression Inventory (BDI)**
BDI was developed in English in 1961 and revised in 1978 (BDI-IA) and 1996 (BDI-II) and it can be utilized both as screening tool and severity measurement in diagnosed patients. A shorter version is available for primary care as screening tool, i.e., the BDI Fast Screen for Medical Patients (BDI-FS). BDI-II is the widely used version. Regarding 21 major depressive symptoms (items), patients are asked to indicate their severity in the last 2 weeks, with a 4-levels Likert-scale ranging from 0 ('symptom absent') to 3 ('severe symptoms') [28, 27].

Summing items scores, a total score ranging from 0 to 63 can be obtained, with higher scores indicating more severe depressive symptoms. As screening, a cut-off of 20 is considered to indicate the presence of depressive symptoms. Indeed, in diagnosed patients, minimal, mild, moderate, and severe depression are identified by score ranges of 0–13, 14–19, 20–28, and above 28, respectively [28, 27].

This version of the scale showed good content and construct validity and good correlation with other validated tools, such as Hamilton Psychiatric Rating Scale Depression (HRSD) and MMPI [27, 28].

It requires 5–10 min to be filled and its scoring is quick, with the possibility to use the scale both for screening and depression severity evaluation in primary and specialty settings [28, 27].

**2. Patients Health Questionnaire (PHQ)**
This scale was developed in English in 1999, to evaluate the presence of symptoms related to several psychiatric disorders in primary care and it showed good diagnostic validity and accuracy [29]. In the following years, selected items of the scale were validated as separate instruments aimed at suggesting a diagnosis of depression or to evaluate its severity, such as PHQ-9. This scale comprises the 9 items of PHQ dedicated to depressive symptoms and patients are asked to indicate how often they experienced symptoms in the last 4 weeks, through a with a 4-levels Likert-scale ranging from 0 ('not at all') to 3 ('nearly every day') [30].

Total score is derived by items' score sum and ranges from 0 to 27 with higher scores indicating more severe depressive symptoms. A severity cut-off of 10 as score was set [30].

PHQ-9 is reliable and valid for screening and severity evaluation in diagnosed patients and could be utilized both in primary care and specialist settings. Moreover, its filling and scoring are quick, and it is widely considered in the literature as a diagnostic test [30, 31].

### 9.2.2.3   Mixed Instruments for Anxiety and Depression

#### 1. Patients Health Questionnaire-4 (PHQ-4)

Another instrument derived from PHQ is PHQ-4, which includes two items from PHQ-9 (i.e., PHQ-2) and two items from GAD-7 (i.e., GAD-2). Therefore, this scale developed in 2010 is a very-brief screening tool for both anxiety and depression, mainly in general population and primary settings. The tool includes core criteria for the diagnosis of depressive and generalized anxiety disorders and its reliability and validity in general population is good [32].

Answer modalities and scoring algorithm are the same as PHQ-9 and GAD-7, with a total possible score ranging from 0 to 12. Cut-off for depression and anxiety disorder screening are evaluated separately for PHQ-2 and the GAD-2, with a total score of 3 for each scale considered as suggestive of probable cases of depression or anxiety, respectively [33, 34].

## 9.2.3   PTSD

Regarding PTSD, it is noteworthy to highlight that PTSD may be different in non-clinical and clinical subjects, i.e., those who experienced major traumas. Therefore, it is advisable to assess PTSD if suspected rather than perform screening for it [35]. However, research about the estimation of its prevalence in primary headache disorder utilizing the described scales is available [36–38].

#### 1. PTSD Checklist-Civilian Version (PCL-C)

PCL-C was developed in English in 1993 to assess PTSD symptoms in acute traumatic injuries population. It is a patient-rated 17-items scale with a 5-levels Likert-scale ranging from 1 ('not at all') to 5 ('extremely'). Patients are asked to indicate how much they have been bothered by described PTSD symptoms without a shared recall period in the literature [39].

Total possible score, which is obtained summing single items' score, ranges 17–85 with higher scores inidcating higher possibility of PTSD, and a score equal or higher than 44 suggesting possible PTSD. This is a very accurate tool to suggest a PTSD diagnosis, it takes about 5–10 min to be filled and it considered in the literature as relatively time-consuming [40].

**2. Primary Care-PTSD Screen (PC-PTSD)**
A less sensitive but quicker assessment, especially for acute PTSD symptoms, is PC-PTSD, that was developed in 2013 and includes four items of the PCL-C. Answer modality is the same as PCL-C and it requires only 1 min to be filled. Selected items include reexperiencing, behavioural avoidance, emotional avoidance, and hyperarousal symptoms. Answering differently form 'not at all' to three out of four items is considered as suggestive of PTSD symptoms, but it is not sufficient to suggest a diagnosis [40].

## 9.3  Clinical Scales to Assess Cognitive Status and Aspects in Pain Processing in Headache and Migraine

**1. Subjective Cognitive Impairments Scale (MIG-SCOG)**
This scale was formulated to provide self-report measures of cognitive dysfunction in migraine patients. The MIG-SCOG was developed to quantify self-reported subjective cognitive symptoms during migraine attacks. It is a brief assessment tool (9-items) which allows to investigate two cognitive domains: executive functions (decreased attention, processing speed, orientation, and planning) and language (naming abilities).

There are three response options ('often', 'sometimes', 'no'), the total score is the sum of the score obtained in the individual items. Score ranges from 0 to 18, and higher values indicate greater impairment of cognitive function [41].

**2. Headache-Specific Locus of Control Scale (HSLC)**
This instrument was designed to assess headache sufferers' beliefs about the factors that influence the development of their condition. HSLC consists of 33 items, with response alternatives on a five-point Likert's Scale from 1 ('strongly disagree') to 5 ('strongly agree').

It includes three subscales: Health Care Professionals locus of control, internal locus of control, and chance locus of control. Total score of HSLC ranges from 33 to 165, with subscales scores that range from 11 to 55 for professional and external locus of control, and from 10 to 50 for internal locus of control [42, 43].

**3. Brief Illness Perception Questionnaire (BIPQ)**
To date, no migraine-specific scales are available to assess cognitive perception of the disease. However, BIPQ is widely used in migraine research, and a sample of headache patients was recruited for its validation. The Brief IPQ is an easy-to-use instrument to assess the cognitive and emotional representations of illness. The BIPQ consist of eight items rated using a 0–10 response scale, plus one open-ended

question. Items assess cognitive illness representations, emotional representations and illness comprehensibility, while the open-ended question assess the causal representation of the illness.

The total score is the sum of the individual item scores, taking into account the reverse-scored items. Higher score reflects a worse perception of the disease [44].

### 4. Pain Catastrophizing Scale (PCS)

PCS is a widely used tool in both clinical practice and research, developed to assess pain catastrophizing in patients with chronic pain. PCS evaluates the mechanisms by which catastrophizing affects the experience of pain. It is a 13-item instrument on a 5-point response scale from 0 ('not at all') to 4 ('all the time'), to investigate rumination, magnification, and helplessness.

Score ranges from 0 to 52, with a cut-off of 30 indicating clinically relevant levels of pain catastrophizing [45].

### 5. Headache Management Self-Efficacy Scale (HMSE)

This instrument was developed from the 51-item Headache Self-efficacy Scale (HSE) to assess the level of confidence in managing headache pain and preventing headache episodes.

It is a patient-rated 25-item scale based on 7-point Likert's scale from 1 ('strongly disagree') to 7 ('strongly agree'). Higher scores indicate better effectiveness in disease management, and better coping skills [46].

### 6. Pain-Coping Inventory (PCI)

This scale was validated in 2003, to assess coping strategies in patients with chronic pain conditions, including migraine. The PCI is easy to administer and time-efficient. It consists of 33 items on a 4-point Likert scale ranging from 1 ('hardly ever') to 4 ('very often').

The total score is the sum of the individual items score, and allows the identification of active (transformation, distraction, and reducing demands) and passive (retreating, worrying, and resting) pain management strategies [47].

## 9.4  Conclusion

Despite the possible shared epidemiology and etiopathogenesis is still widely unknown, primary headache patients may often present also psychiatric disorders or cognitive impairment. In order to optimize the treatment, a deeper evaluation of the epidemiology of this phenomenon and possible presenting phenotype is needed. In clinical practice, the awareness of the co-existence of these conditions is fundamental to ensure holistic care management. Therefore, the use of shared and accurate evaluation instruments psychiatric disorders and cognitive impairment is recommended in primary headache patients. When choosing an instrument for clinical practice or research, its content and accuracy features should be considered, along with its appropriateness for our aim, target population, development setting, and research comparability.

# References


1. Haut SR, Bigal ME, Lipton RB. Chronic disorders with episodic manifestations: focus on epilepsy and migraine. Lancet Neurol. 2006;5(2):148–57. https://doi.org/10.1016/s1474-4422(06)70348-9.
2. Caponnetto V, Deodato M, Robotti M, Koutsokera M, Pozzilli V, Galati C, et al. Comorbidities of primary headache disorders: a literature review with meta-analysis. J Headache Pain. 2021;22(1):71. https://doi.org/10.1186/s10194-021-01281-z.
3. Burch RC, Buse DC, Lipton RB. Migraine: epidemiology, burden, and comorbidity. Neurol Clin. 2019;37(4):631–49. https://doi.org/10.1016/j.ncl.2019.06.001.
4. Bag B, Hacihasanoglu R, Tufekci FG. Examination of anxiety, hostility and psychiatric disorders in patients with migraine and tension-type headache. Int J Clin Pract. 2005;59(5):515–21. https://doi.org/10.1111/j.1368-5031.2005.00522.x.
5. Giri S, Tronvik EA, Hagen K. The bidirectional temporal relationship between headache and affective disorders: longitudinal data from the HUNT studies. J Headache Pain. 2022;23(1):14. https://doi.org/10.1186/s10194-022-01388-x.
6. Dresler T, Caratozzolo S, Guldolf K, Huhn JI, Loiacono C, Niiberg-Pikksööt T, et al. Understanding the nature of psychiatric comorbidity in migraine: a systematic review focused on interactions and treatment implications. J Headache Pain. 2019;20(1):51. https://doi.org/10.1186/s10194-019-0988-x.
7. Vuralli D, Ayata C, Bolay H. Cognitive dysfunction and migraine 17 psychology and cognitive sciences 1701 psychology 11 medical and health sciences 1103 clinical sciences 11 medical and health sciences 1109 neurosciences. J Headache Pain. 2018;19(1) https://doi.org/10.1186/s10194-018-0933-4.
8. Radat F, Lantéri-Minet M, Nachit-Ouinekh F, Massiou H, Lucas C, Pradalier A, et al. The GRIM2005 study of migraine consultation in France. III: Psychological features of subjects with migraine. Cephalalgia. 2009;29(3):338–50. https://doi.org/10.1111/j.1468-2982.2008.01718.x.
9. Seng EK, Buse DC, Klepper JE, Mayson SJ, Grinberg AS, Grosberg BM, et al. Psychological factors associated with chronic migraine and severe migraine-related disability: an observational study in a tertiary headache center. Headache. 2017;57(4):593–604. https://doi.org/10.1111/head.13021.
10. Boynton PM, Greenhalgh T. Selecting, designing, and developing your questionnaire. BMJ (Clin Res Ed). 2004;328(7451):1312–5. https://doi.org/10.1136/bmj.328.7451.1312.
11. Floyd AE, Gupta V. Minnesota multiphasic personality inventory. Treasure Island, FL: StatPearl; 2022.
12. Tellegen A, Ben-Porath YS. The new uniform T scores for the MMPI—2: Rationale, derivation, and appraisal. Psychol Assess. 1992;4(2):145–55. https://doi.org/10.1037/1040-3590.4.2.145.
13. Naylor B, Boag S, Gustin SM. New evidence for a pain personality? A critical review of the last 120 years of pain and personality. Scand J Pain. 2017;17:58–67. https://doi.org/10.1016/j.sjpain.2017.07.011.
14. Schenck LA, Andrasik F. Behavioral and psychological aspects of cluster headache: an overview. Neurol Sci. 2019;40(Suppl 1):3–7. https://doi.org/10.1007/s10072-019-03831-5.
15. Sheehan DV, Lecrubier Y, Sheehan KH, Amorim P, Janavs J, Weiller E, et al. The Mini-International Neuropsychiatric Interview (M.I.N.I.): the development and validation of a structured diagnostic psychiatric interview for DSM-IV and ICD-10. J Clin Psychiatry. 1998;59(Suppl 20):22–33. Quiz 4–57
16. Gaynes BN, DeVeaugh-Geiss J, Weir S, Gu H, MacPherson C, Schulberg HC, et al. Feasibility and diagnostic validity of the M-3 checklist: a brief, self-rated screen for depressive, bipolar, anxiety, and post-traumatic stress disorders in primary care. Ann Fam Med. 2010;8(2):160. https://doi.org/10.1370/afm.1092.
17. Driessen MT, Cohen JM, Thompson SF, Patterson-Lomba O, Seminerio MJ, Carr K, et al. Real-world effectiveness after initiating fremanezumab treatment in US patients with episodic

and chronic migraine or difficult-to-treat migraine. J Headache Pain. 2022;23(1):56. https://doi.org/10.1186/s10194-022-01415-x.

18. Esmael A, Abdelsalam M, Shoukri A, Elsherif M. Subjective cognitive impairment in patients with transformed migraine and the associated psychological and sleep disturbances. Sleep Breath. 2021;25(4):2119–26. https://doi.org/10.1007/s11325-021-02308-0.

19. Bougea A, Spantideas N, Galanis P, Katsika P, Boufidou F, Voskou P, et al. Salivary inflammatory markers in tension type headache and migraine: the SalHead cohort study. Neurol Sci. 2020;41(4):877–84. https://doi.org/10.1007/s10072-019-04151-4.

20. Guner D, Eyigor C. Efficacy of ultrasound-guided greater occipital nerve pulsed radiofrequency therapy in chronic refractory migraine. Acta Neurol Belg. 2022; https://doi.org/10.1007/s13760-022-01972-7.

21. Cappon D, Ryterska A, Akram H, Lagrata S, Cheema S, Hyam J, et al. The sensitivity to change of the cluster headache quality of life scale assessed before and after deep brain stimulation of the ventral tegmental area. J Headache Pain. 2021;22(1):52. https://doi.org/10.1186/s10194-021-01251-5.

22. Pohl H, Streit AC, Neumeier MS, Merki-Feld GS, Ruch W, Gantenbein AR. Migraine and happiness. Womens Health Rep (New Rochelle, NY). 2022;3(1):155–61. https://doi.org/10.1089/whr.2021.0122.

23. Spitzer RL, Kroenke K, Williams JB, Löwe B. A brief measure for assessing generalized anxiety disorder: the GAD-7. Arch Intern Med. 2006;166(10):1092–7. https://doi.org/10.1001/archinte.166.10.1092.

24. Donker T, van Straten A, Marks I, Cuijpers P. Quick and easy self-rating of generalized anxiety disorder: validity of the Dutch web-based GAD-7, GAD-2 and GAD-SI. Psychiatry Res. 2011;188(1):58–64. https://doi.org/10.1016/j.psychres.2011.01.016.

25. Beck AT, Epstein N, Brown G, Steer RA. An inventory for measuring clinical anxiety: psychometric properties. J Consult Clin Psychol. 1988;56(6):893–7. https://doi.org/10.1037/0022-006X.56.6.893.

26. Lichtenberg PA. Handbook of assessment in clinical gerontology. San Diego: Academic Press; 2010.

27. Beck AT, Steer RA, Carbin MG. Psychometric properties of the Beck Depression Inventory: Twenty-five years of evaluation. Clin Psychol Rev. 1988;8(1):77–100. https://doi.org/10.1016/0272-7358(88)90050-5.

28. Jackson-Koku G. Beck depression inventory. Occup Med. 2016;66(2):174–5. https://doi.org/10.1093/occmed/kqv087.

29. Spitzer RL, Kroenke K, Williams JB, Group PHQPCS. Validation and utility of a self-report version of PRIME-MD: the PHQ primary care study. JAMA. 1999;282(18):1737–44.

30. Negeri ZF, Levis B, Sun Y, He C, Krishnan A, Wu Y, et al. Accuracy of the Patient Health Questionnaire-9 for screening to detect major depression: updated systematic review and individual participant data meta-analysis. BMJ (Clin Res Ed). 2021;375:n2183. https://doi.org/10.1136/bmj.n2183.

31. Muñoz-Navarro R, Cano-Vindel A, Medrano LA, Schmitz F, Ruiz-Rodríguez P, Abellán-Maeso C, et al. Utility of the PHQ-9 to identify major depressive disorder in adult patients in Spanish primary care centres. BMC Psychiatry. 2017;17(1):291. https://doi.org/10.1186/s12888-017-1450-8.

32. Löwe B, Wahl I, Rose M, Spitzer C, Glaesmer H, Wingenfeld K, et al. A 4-item measure of depression and anxiety: validation and standardization of the Patient Health Questionnaire-4 (PHQ-4) in the general population. J Affect Disord. 2010;122(1–2):86–95. https://doi.org/10.1016/j.jad.2009.06.019.

33. Kroenke K, Spitzer RL, Williams JB. The Patient Health Questionnaire-2: validity of a two-item depression screener. Med Care. 2003;41(11):1284–92.

34. Löwe B, Kroenke K, Gräfe K. Detecting and monitoring depression with a two-item questionnaire (PHQ-2). J Psychosom Res. 2005;58(2):163–71.

35. Conybeare D, Behar E, Solomon A, Newman MG, Borkovec T. The PTSD checklist—civilian version: reliability, validity, and factor structure in a nonclinical sample. J Clin Psychol. 2012;68(6):699–713.
36. Peterlin BL, Tietjen G, Meng S, Lidicker J, Bigal M. Post-traumatic stress disorder in episodic and chronic migraine. Headache. 2008;48(4):517–22. https://doi.org/10.1111/j.1526-4610.2008.00917.x.
37. de Leeuw R, Schmidt JE, Carlson CR. Traumatic stressors and post-traumatic stress disorder symptoms in headache patients. Headache. 2005;45(10):1365–74. https://doi.org/10.1111/j.1526-4610.2005.00269.x.
38. Zarei MR, Shabani M, Chamani G, Abareghi F, Razavinasab M, Nazeri M. Migraine patients have a higher prevalence of PTSD symptoms in comparison to chronic tension-type headache and healthy subjects: a case-control study. Acta Odontol Scand. 2016;74(8):633–5. https://doi.org/10.1080/00016357.2016.1232435.
39. Weathers FW, Litz BT, Herman DS, Huska JA, Keane TM, editors. The PTSD Checklist (PCL): Reliability, validity, and diagnostic utility. In: Annual convention of the International Society for Traumatic Stress Studies, San Antonio, TX; 1993.
40. Hanley J, Deroon-Cassini T, Brasel K. Efficiency of a four-item posttraumatic stress disorder screen in trauma patients. J Trauma Acute Care Surg. 2013;75(4):722–7. https://doi.org/10.1097/TA.0b013e3182a53a5f.
41. Gil-Gouveia R, Oliveira AG, Martins IP. A subjective cognitive impairment scale for migraine attacks. the MIG-SCOG: Development and validation. Cephalalgia. 2011;31(9):984–91. https://doi.org/10.1177/0333102411408359.
42. Martin NJ, Holroyd KA, Penzien DB. The headache-specific locus of control scale: adaptation to recurrent headaches. Headache J Head Face Pain. 1990;30(11):729–34. https://doi.org/10.1111/j.1526-4610.1990.hed3011729.x.
43. Heath RL, Saliba M, Mahmassani O, Major SC, Khoury BA. Locus of control moderates the relationship between headache pain and depression. J Headache Pain. 2008;9(5):301–8. https://doi.org/10.1007/s10194-008-0055-5.
44. Broadbent E, Petrie KJ, Main J, Weinman J. The brief illness perception questionnaire. J Psychosom Res. 2006;60(6):631–7. https://doi.org/10.1016/j.jpsychores.2005.10.020.
45. Sullivan MJL, Bishop SR, Pivik J. The pain catastrophizing scale: development and validation. Psychol Assess. 1995;7(4):524–32. https://doi.org/10.1037/1040-3590.7.4.524.
46. French DJ, Holroyd KA, Pinell C, Malinoski PT, O'Donnell F, Hill KR. Perceived self-efficacy and headache-related disability. Headache. 2000;40(8):647–56. https://doi.org/10.1046/j.1526-4610.2000.040008647.x.
47. Kraaimaat FW, Evers AWM. Pain-coping strategies in chronic pain patients: psychometric characteristics of the Pain-Coping Inventory (PCI). Int J Behav Med. 2003;10(4):343–63. https://doi.org/10.1207/S15327558IJBM1004_5.

# Chapter 10
# Clinical Instruments for Treatment Monitoring and Optimization in Headache and Migraine

Sait Ashina and Amanda Macone

## 10.1 Introduction

Headache is the most prevalent neurological disorder in the population, and one of the most widespread pain-related and disabling conditions worldwide [1–3]. Migraine and tension-type headache (TTH) are the most common primary headache disorders in the general population [4, 5]. Headache disorders, including migraine and TTH, are commonly diagnosed and managed by neurologists, but primary care physicians, family physicians and other specialists may also be involved in headache management [6]. In a recent population-based study from the United States, The ObserVational survey of the Epidemiology, tReatment and Care of MigrainE (OVERCOME) [7], patients were most likely to have at least one lifetime medical consultation for headache/migraine with primary care provider (70.3%), followed by consultation in a neurology clinic (28.1%), or with a headache specialist (15.6%).

Effective acute treatment can improve or decrease the pain, associated symptoms, and disability associated with headache or migraine attack [8, 9]. Preventative treatment can reduce the frequency of headache/migraine attacks and headache days, improve headache-related disability and impact, and prevent the development

S. Ashina (✉)
BIDMC Comprehensive Headache Center, Department of Neurology and Department of Anesthesia, Critical Care and Pain Medicine, Harvard Medical School, Beth Israel Deaconess Medical Center, Boston, MA, USA

Department of Clinical Medicine, Faculty of Health Sciences, University of Copenhagen, Copenhagen, Denmark
e-mail: sait.ashina@bidmc.harvard.edu

A. Macone
BIDMC Comprehensive Headache Center, Department of Neurology and Department of Anesthesia, Critical Care and Pain Medicine, Harvard Medical School, Beth Israel Deaconess Medical Center, Boston, MA, USA



P. Yalınay Dikmen, A. Özge (eds.), *Clinical Scales for Headache Disorders*, Headache, https://doi.org/10.1007/978-3-031-25938-8_10

**Table 10.1** Clinical instruments for treatment assessment, monitoring and optimization in headache and migraine

| Generic/non-specific | Migraine specific |
| --- | --- |
| Headache Under Response to Treatment (HURT) Questionnaire | Migraine Assessment of Current Therapy (Migraine-ACT) |
| Medication Dependence Questionnaire in Headache (MDQ-H) | Migraine Treatment Optimization Questionnaire (MTOQ) |
| Treatment Satisfaction Questionnaire for Medication (TSQM) | Patient Perception of Migraine Questionnaire Revised (PPMQ-R) |
| Screener and Opioid Assessment for Patients with Pain Revised (SOAPP-R) | Migraine Therapy Assessment Questionnaire (MTAQ) |
| Current Opioid Misuse Measure (COMM) | Migraine Prevention Questionnaire (MPQ-5) |
|  | Migraine Completeness of Response Survey (CORS) |
|  | Migraine Treatment Satisfaction Measure (MTSM) |

of medication overuse headache [9, 10]. Individuals with migraine may have specific expectations and preferences about their acute or preventive treatment. They may except or wish for rapid and complete headache relief, consistent headache relief, ability to return to normal functioning, improvement or relief of migraine-associated symptoms, reduction in headache frequency or recurrence, and minimal adverse effects associated with treatment [11, 12]. Treatment response is the most important key element for the assessment and optimization of a therapy given to patients, and assists in measuring the efficacy of pharmacological or device treatments in headache and migraine management. Several patient-reported outcomes and self-reported measures may be used for that purpose [13, 14]. They can be divided into generic or migraine-specific instruments (Table 10.1). Generic instruments include the Headache Under Response to Treatment (HURT) Questionnaire [15, 16], Medication Dependence Questionnaire in Headache (MDQ-H) [17], Treatment Satisfaction Questionnaire for Medication (TSQM) [18], Screener and Opioid Assessment for Patients with Pain Revised (SOAPP-R) [19, 20], and Current Opioid Misuse Measure (COMM) [21].

Migraine-specific instruments which measure optimization of, and/or satisfaction with, acute and preventive medications include the Migraine Assessment of Current Therapy (Migraine-ACT) [22–24], Migraine Treatment Optimization Questionnaire (MTOQ) [25, 26], Patient Perception of Migraine Questionnaire Revised (PPMQ-R) [27], Migraine Therapy Assessment Questionnaire (MTAQ) [28], Migraine Prevention Questionnaire (MPQ-5) [29], Migraine Completeness of Response Survey (CORS) [30], and Migraine Treatment Satisfaction Measure (MTSM) [31, 32].

## 10.2  Generic Instruments

### 10.2.1  *Headache Under Response to Treatment (HURT) Questionnaire*

The HURT questionnaire is a treatment outcome measure which was developed to specifically help guide primary care physicians in the management of patients with headache [15, 16, 33]. This questionnaire was developed by the working group, Lifting The Burden (LTB), a nongovernmental organization working in official relations with the World Health Organization (WHO), to direct the Global Campaign against Headache [34]. The HURT questionnaire is an 8-item, self-administered questionnaire assessing headache frequency, disability, medication use and effect, patients' perceptions of headache "control", and knowledge/understanding of the diagnosis. The first seven questions in the HURT have five categorical response options, which are graded from good to bad. Question 8 has dichotomous response option: yes/no. The responses are numerically coded and summed to the total score, which ranges from 0 to 24 with a higher score indicating a high headache burden. However, the questions also address heterogeneous concepts related to headache care and treatment outcome, and may provide more information when analyzed separately. For instance, HURT also aims to guide management not only by indicating when treatment is or is not optimal, but also by suggesting how management should be modified to improve outcome. This can assist the treating physician with clinical advice and decision making.

Previous studies have demonstrated that HURT is reliable and functions comparably across various headache conditions [15, 16, 33, 35, 36]. Moreover, HUNT has been shown to correlate with other validated scales and measures, such as the Migraine Disability Assessment Scale (MIDAS), the Headache Impact Test (HIT-6), the Patient Health Questionnaire (PHQ-9), health-related quality of life measure (HRQoL v2), and the Migraine Prevention Questionnaire (MPQ). HURT scores correlated positively with (MPQ), an instrument indicating the need for preventative pharmacological treatment of migraine [15]. The psychometric evaluation of HURT revealed a two-factor model: (1) headache frequency, disability and medication use; and (2) medication efficacy and headache control items [16]. In addition, responses could be categorized into three areas: white (no action needed), lightly shaded (action suggested), and darker shading (action required) [15].

### 10.2.2  *Medication Dependence Questionnaire in Headache*

MDQ-H has been developed to measure dependence on analgesics and on migraine attack treatments in patients with headache. The questionnaire is based on the definitions of substance dependence contained in the fourth edition of the Diagnostic and Statistical Manual of Mental Disorders (DSM-IV) criteria [17]. The MDQ-H is a self-administered questionnaire containing 21 questions that involve each diagnostic criterion of dependence described in the DSM-IV. For each item, patients are asked to describe their medication consumption according to a 7-point Likert scale (1: never or not at all; 3: sometimes or a little; 5: often or quite a lot; and 7: always or completely). Total score was obtained by adding the scores for all the items. A high total score means an important disturbance in the way the patient uses his or her medication for the treatment of headache. Patients with chronic migraine and medication overuse headache have been found to have higher MDQ-H scores than patients with episodic migraine [37, 38].

Higher MDQ-H scores have also been shown to predict the relapse of medication overuse headache within 12 months after either an inpatient or outpatient withdrawal procedure in patients with medication overuse headache [38]. The global MDQ-H score has also been shown to predict the number of days of medication use, the number of days of headache, and emotional distress [17]. Moreover, MDQ-H scores were reported to be higher for patients with a headache associated with chronic substance use, than for patients with migraine and TTH [17]. However, criticism of MDQ-H has been raised. It has been argued that the questionnaire only measures the dimension of dependence and does not provide a cut-off on which patients should be considered to have medication overuse headache, and maybe more difficult to administer in primary and tertiary care settings [39].

### 10.2.3 Treatment Satisfaction Questionnaire for Medication (TSQM)

Treatment satisfaction is an important aspect of patient management. It is defined as the patient's evaluation of important attributes associated with the process and outcomes of the treatment experience [27, 40]. TSQM is a 14-item, generic measure of satisfaction with treatment, and can also be applied to patients with migraine [18, 41, 42]. TSQM contains four domains with different questions regarding effectiveness, side effects, convenience, and global satisfaction. The scores range from 0 to 100, with higher scores representative of higher satisfaction.

### 10.2.4 Screener and Opioid Assessment for Patients with Pain Revised

Opioid use in migraine or other types of primary headaches is typically discouraged. However, previous population-based surveys have found it to be common, and associated with negative consequences such as higher health care costs for patients with migraine, increased risk of transformation from episodic to chronic migraine, and more severe headache-related disability, symptomology, comorbidities, and greater healthcare resource utilization for headache [43–46].

SOAPP-R is a 24-item, self-report measure and screener tool for health care providers and clinicians. It assists in the assessment of aberrant medication-related behaviors in patients with chronic pain, including refractory chronic migraine, and to determine how much monitoring of opioid therapy is needed [19, 20, 47]. SOAPP-R is a revised and updated version of the original SOAPP questionnaire, which was developed based on expert consensus [19, 48]. SOAPP-R asks patients to rate the frequency of occurrence using a Likert scale that ranges from 0 to 4 (0 = "never," 1 = "seldom," 2 = "sometimes," 3 = "often," 4 = "very often"). A patient's total score is calculated by summing the scores of the individual items. Total score ranges from 0 to 96, with higher score indicating higher risk for opioid misuse. A score of $\geq 18$ indicates high risk for opioid misuse. SOAPP-R has been validated and cross-validated, and shown to have a good internal reliability, specificity, and sensitivity in identifying patients at elevated risk for opioid misuse [19, 49]. Disadvantages of SOAPP-R include the possible risk of misleading and false responses, and impracticality in clinical settings [50].

### 10.2.5   Current Opioid Misuse Measure

The COMM is a brief, self-report measure to monitor patients with chronic pain who are prescribed opioids [51]. This measure assesses aberrant medication-related behaviors in the past 30 days. Aberrant medication-related behaviors are defined as behaviors that are relating to addiction, or taking a medication in a way other than how it is prescribed [51, 52]. The COMM was developed with the assistance of pain and addiction experts as well as advise from practicing pain management specialists. The excellent internal consistency and test-retest reliability of COMM has been demonstrated [21, 51]. The responses are rated on a Likert scale that ranges from 0 to 4 (0 = "never," 1 = "seldom," 2 = "sometimes," 3 = "often," 4 = "very often"). The measure has 17 items which are summed to create a total score. A total score of 9 or higher is considered to be a positive screen for opioid misuse.

## 10.3   Migraine-Specific Instruments

### 10.3.1   Migraine Assessment of Current Therapy

The 4-item Migraine-ACT Questionnaire is a brief assessment tool, developed with input from international headache experts, to identify patients needing a change in acute migraine treatment in the primary care setting [23, 24, 53]. The questionnaire has demonstrated excellent reliability and validity, and can be used on the return or follow-up visit to evaluate the effectiveness of acute treatment [22, 24]. It includes the 4 following domains: headache impact, global assessment of relief, consistency of treatment response, and emotional response to treatment. The questions are, "When you take your treatment": (1) "Does the headache pain disappear within 2 hours?", (2) "Are you able to function normally within 2 hours?", (3) "Does your migraine medication work consistently in the majority of the attacks?", and (4) "Are you comfortable enough with your medication to be able to plan your daily activities?" [23]. Scoring is done by summing the "yes" scores. The total Migraine-ACT score ranges from 0 to 4. A total score $\leq 2$ indicates the need for a change in acute migraine therapy. The change in Migraine-ACT score has been shown to correlate with changes in SF-36, MIDAS, and MTAQ scores [24]. It has been suggested that the Migraine-ACT can be used more reliably than the MIDAS questionnaire for detecting improvements in treatment response in patients with migraine [54].

## 10.3.2  *Migraine Treatment Optimization Questionnaire*

The original mTOQ was developed to help health care providers and clinicians assess and optimize acute migraine treatment [8, 25, 26]. The mTOQ has been validated in five languages and several versions of length. Initially, a 15-item (mTOQ-15) and five-item (mTOQ-5) self-administered questionnaires were derived and validated [25]. The authors of this initial study suggested to use mTOQ-15 in research, and mTOQ-5 in primary care. The original validation studies of the mTOQ used dichotomous "yes" or "no" response options. In the American Migraine Prevalence and Prevention (AMPP) study, categorical response options were given for 6 mTOQ questions, which assessed the optimization of acute treatment in persons with migraine [26]. Thus, in mTOQ-6, responses to each item scored as: never = 1, rarely = 2, less than half the time = 3, or half the time or more = 4. The mTOQ-6 total score can be calculated by summing the score for each question (total score range of 6–24 points), with a higher score indicative of better acute migraine treatment optimization. The questions in the mTOQ-6 focus on how often respondents have the following outcomes after acute migraine treatment: return to normal function, 2-hour pain free, sustained 24-hour pain relief, tolerability, comfortable making plans, and perceived control [26]. After additional validation, from 4 items from the mTOQ-6 were selected to better assess acute treatment efficacy and to eliminate redundancies. This led to the creation of the mTOQ-4, which was developed and tested in the migraine population [55]. Survey response options of mTOQ-4 are: never = 0, rarely = 0, half the time = 1, $\geq$ half the time = 2. Total sum scores range from 0 to 8.

The authors defined four categorizes of treatment efficacy: very poor treatment efficacy (total score of 0), poor treatment efficacy (total score of 1–5), moderate treatment efficacy (total score of 6–7), and maximum treatment efficacy (total score of 8). The mTOQ-4 has been found to be useful in both clinical and population-based studies [55]. When measured with mTOQ-4, ineffective acute migraine treatment was shown to be a risk factor for transformation of migraine from episodic to chronic form [55].

### 10.3.3   Patient Perception of Migraine Questionnaire Revised

The 15-item Patient Perception of Migraine Questionnaire (PPMQ) was one of the few disease-specific questionnaires developed to assess patient satisfaction with acute migraine treatment [56]. It was found to be a valid and reliable measurement of patient perception regarding drug attributes in relation to the acute treatment of symptoms associated with migraine [56]. The revised version of PPMQ, PPMQ-R, added measures important to patients, such as convenience and ease of use of medication, treatment effect on functional ability, and side effects [27, 40].

### 10.3.4   Migraine Therapy Assessment Questionnaire

The MTAQ was developed based on expert opinion, advice from patient focus groups, and previous work in diseases such as asthma [28, 57]. MTAQ is a 9-item questionnaire assessing migraine treatment, and includes questions on symptom control, attack frequency, knowledge/behavior barriers, economic burden, and overall patient satisfaction with migraine treatment [28, 58]. MTAQ was proven to be reliable and valid, and is able to identify migraine patients with suboptimal treatment in a primary and tertiary care setting [28, 59]. Each item in the questionnaire receives a "yes" = 1 or "no" = 0 score, except for questions 1, 2, 5, and 9, which are inversely coded with a "no" response score of 1 [28]. Moreover, questions 3 and 4 are scored together, and scoring of these questions is described in detail by Chatterton et al. [28].

### 10.3.5   Migraine Prevention Questionnaire

The MPQ was developed by Lipton et al. [29] to help clinicians assess treatment needs in migraine patients, and consider the initiation of preventative pharmacological treatments. This questionnaire underwent psychometric testing and was shown to be reliable with good validity [14, 16, 29]. The 5-item questionnaire assesses the headache frequency, use of acute migraine treatment, headache related impairment, as well as anxiety related to headache. The total score is the sum of responses to individual items [14]. The total score falls into one of three categories: (1) preventive treatment not indicated, (2) consider preventive treatment, and (3) offer preventive treatment. It has been demonstrated that MPQ scores positively correlate with scores from HURT, a non-specific measure developed to help and guide primary care physicians to manage patients with headache [16, 29].

### 10.3.6 Migraine Completeness of Response Survey

Migraine Completeness of Response Survey (CORS) has been developed to measure the completeness of response associated with a single migraine treatment, and for the comparison of response between different treatments [30]. The survey was designed with advice from interviews with focus groups including migraine patients and headache specialists. In the final version, CORS included 32 items. 24 of the 32 items focus on the performance of individual treatments, and 8 items allow for comparison between 2 treatments. The questionnaire addresses five concepts concerning migraine treatment: frequency of complete relief, speed of complete relief, speed of return to functionality, frequency of migraine recurrence, and confidence in migraine treatment [30]. The scoring of CORS is described in detail by Coon et al. [30].

Higher scores indicate better response to the medication. The advantage of CORS is that it can allow for a head-to-head comparison of migraine treatments.

### 10.3.7 Migraine Treatment Satisfaction Measure

MTSM is a migraine-specific measure which was developed for the assessment of satisfaction with treatment [31, 32]. It is comprised of four parts, assessing treatment-related concerns communicated by patients: (part 1) expectations about treatment outcomes; (part 2) importance rankings of nine attributes (pain relief, speed of relief, freedom from pain, additional symptoms, confidence in treatment, disruption in life, dosing, freedom from relapse, and ease of use); (part 3) report of treatment outcome; (part 4) patient satisfaction with the treatment [31, 32]. Scoring is complicated, and involves five steps which are described in detail by Martin et al. [31]. The total MTSM score characterizes patient expectations and satisfaction about their treatment. MTSM scores have been shown to be associated with Migraine Symptom Frequency Bother scores, MIDAS general health, mental health, and vitality subscales of SF-36 [60].

## 10.4 Conclusions

There are several generic and migraine-specific instruments that measure treatment outcomes. The instruments can be important to understanding the effectiveness and need for migraine treatments.

# References


1. Collaborators GUND. Burden of neurological disorders across the US from 1990-2017: a global burden of disease study. JAMA Neurol. 2021;78(2):165–76.
2. Deuschl G, Beghi E, Fazekas F, Varga T, Christoforidi KA, Sipido E, et al. The burden of neurological diseases in Europe: an analysis for the Global Burden of Disease Study 2017. Lancet Public Health. 2020;5(10):e551–e67.
3. Leonardi M, Grazzi L, D'Amico D, Martelletti P, Guastafierro E, Toppo C, et al. Global burden of headache disorders in children and adolescents 2007-2017. Int J Environ Res Public Health. 2020;18(1)
4. Ashina M. Migraine. N Engl J Med. 2020;383(19):1866–76.
5. Ashina S, Mitsikostas DD, Lee MJ, Yamani N, Wang SJ, Messina R, et al. Tension-type headache. Nat Rev Dis Primers. 2021;7(1):24.
6. Robbins MS. Diagnosis and management of headache: a review. JAMA. 2021;325(18):1874–85.
7. Lipton RB, Nicholson RA, Reed ML, Araujo Andre B, Jaffe DH, Faries DE, et al. Diagnosis, consultation, treatment, and impact of migraine in the US: Results of the OVERCOME (US) study. Headache J Head Face Pain. 2022;62(2):122–40.
8. Eigenbrodt AK, Ashina H, Khan S, Diener H-C, Mitsikostas DD, Sinclair AJ, et al. Diagnosis and management of migraine in ten steps. Nat Rev Neurol. 2021;17(8):501–14.
9. Ailani J, Burch RC, Robbins MS, the Board of Directors of the American Headache Society. The American Headache Society Consensus Statement: Update on integrating new migraine treatments into clinical practice. Headache J Head Face Pain. 2021;61(7):1021–39.
10. Ashina S, Terwindt GM, Steiner TJ, Lee MJ, Porreca F, Tassorelli C, Schwedt TJ, Jensen RH, Diener HC, Lipton RB. Medication overuse headache. Nat Rev Dis Primers. 2023;2;9(1):5. https://doi.org/10.1038/s41572-022-00415-0. PMID: 36732518.
11. Lipton RB, Hamelsky SW, Dayno JM. What do patients with migraine want from acute migraine treatment? Headache. 2002;42(Suppl 1):3–9.
12. Davies GM, Santanello N, Lipton R. Determinants of patient satisfaction with migraine therapy. Cephalalgia. 2000;20(6):554–60.
13. Haywood KL, Mars TS, Potter R, Patel S, Matharu M, Underwood M. Assessing the impact of headaches and the outcomes of treatment: A systematic review of patient-reported outcome measures (PROMs). Cephalalgia. 2018;38(7):1374–86.
14. Buse DC, Rupnow MF, Lipton RB. Assessing and managing all aspects of migraine: migraine attacks, migraine-related functional impairment, common comorbidities, and quality of life. Mayo Clin Proc. 2009;84(5):422–35.
15. Buse DC, Sollars CM, Steiner TJ, Jensen RH, Al Jumah MA, Lipton RB. Why HURT? A review of clinical instruments for headache management. Curr Pain Headache Rep. 2012;16(3):237–54.
16. Steiner TJ, Buse DC, Al Jumah M, Westergaard ML, Jensen RH, Reed ML, et al. The headache under-response to treatment (HURT) questionnaire, an outcome measure to guide follow-up in primary care: development, psychometric evaluation and assessment of utility. J Headache Pain. 2018;19(1):15.
17. Radat F, Irachabal S, Lafittau M, Creac'h C, Dousset V, Henry P. Construction of a Medication Dependence Questionnaire in Headache Patients (MDQ-H) validation of the French version. Headache J Head Face Pain. 2006;46(2):233–9.
18. Atkinson MJ, Sinha A, Hass SL, Colman SS, Kumar RN, Brod M, et al. Validation of a general measure of treatment satisfaction, the Treatment Satisfaction Questionnaire for Medication (TSQM), using a national panel study of chronic disease. Health Qual Life Outcomes. 2004;2:12.
19. Butler SF, Fernandez K, Benoit C, Budman SH, Jamison RN. Validation of the revised Screener and Opioid Assessment for Patients with Pain (SOAPP-R). J Pain. 2008;9(4):360–72.

20. Finkelman MD, Smits N, Kulich RJ, Zacharoff KL, Magnuson BE, Chang H, et al. Development of Short-Form Versions of the Screener and Opioid Assessment for Patients with Pain-Revised (SOAPP-R): a proof-of-principle study. Pain Med. 2017;18(7):1292–302.
21. Butler SF, Budman SH, Fanciullo GJ, Jamison RN. Cross validation of the current opioid misuse measure to monitor chronic pain patients on opioid therapy. Clin J Pain. 2010;26(9):770–6.
22. Dowson AJ, D'Amico D, Tepper SJ, Baos V, Baudet F, Kilminster S. Identifying patients who require a change in their current acute migraine treatment: the Migraine Assessment of Current Therapy (Migraine-ACT) questionnaire. Neurol Sci. 2004;25(Suppl 3):S276–8.
23. Dowson AJ, Tepper SJ, Baos V, Baudet F, D'Amico D, Kilminster S. Identifying patients who require a change in their current acute migraine treatment: the Migraine Assessment of Current Therapy (Migraine-ACT) questionnaire. Curr Med Res Opin. 2004;20(7):1125–35.
24. Kilminster SG, Dowson AJ, Tepper SJ, Baos V, Baudet F, D'Amico D. Reliability, validity, and clinical utility of the migraine-ACT questionnaire. Headache. 2006;46(4):553–62.
25. Lipton RB, Kolodner K, Bigal ME, Valade D, Láinez MJA, Pascual J, et al. Validity and reliability of the Migraine-Treatment Optimization Questionnaire. Cephalalgia. 2009;29(7):751–9.
26. Serrano D, Buse DC, Manack Adams A, Reed ML, Lipton RB. Acute treatment optimization in episodic and chronic migraine: results of the American Migraine Prevalence and Prevention (AMPP) Study. Headache. 2015;55(4):502–18.
27. Revicki DA, Kimel M, Beusterien K, Kwong JW, Varner JA, Ames MH, et al. Validation of the Revised Patient Perception of Migraine Questionnaire: measuring satisfaction with acute migraine treatment. Headache J Head Face Pain. 2006;46(2):240–52.
28. Chatterton ML, Lofland JH, Shechter A, Curtice WS, Hu XH, Lenow J, et al. Reliability and validity of the migraine therapy assessment questionnaire. Headache. 2002;42(10):1006–15.
29. Lipton RB, Serrano D, Buse D, Rupnow MFT, Reed ML, Bigal ME. The Migraine Prevention Questionnaire (MPQ): development and validation [abstract F48]. Headache. 2007;47(5):770–1.
30. Coon CD, Fehnel SE, Davis KH, Runken MC, Beach ME, Cady RK. The development of a survey to measure completeness of response to migraine therapy. Headache. 2012;52(4):550–72.
31. Martin ML, Patrick DL, Bushnell DM, Gandra SR, Gilchrist K. Further validation of an individualized migraine treatment satisfaction measure. Value Health. 2008;11(5):904–12.
32. Patrick DL, Martin ML, Bushnell DM, Pesa J. Measuring satisfaction with migraine treatment: expectations, importance, outcomes, and global ratings. Clin Ther. 2003;25(11):2920–35.
33. Westergaard ML, Steiner TJ, MacGregor EA, Antonaci F, Tassorelli C, Buse DC, et al. The Headache Under-Response to Treatment (HURT) Questionnaire: assessment of utility in headache specialist care. Cephalalgia. 2013;33(4):245–55.
34. Steiner TJ. Lifting the burden: The global campaign against headache. Lancet Neurol. 2004;3(4):204–5.
35. Al Jumah M, Al Khathaami A, Tamim H, Al Owayed A, Kojan S, Jawhary A, et al. HURT (headache under-response to treatment) questionnaire in the management of primary headache disorders: reliability, validity and clinical utility of the Arabic version. J Headache Pain. 2013;14(1):16.
36. Mouaanaki SA, Carlsen LN, Bendtsen L, Jensen RH, Schytz HW. Treatment experiences and clinical characteristics in migraine and tension-type headache patients before the first visit to a tertiary headache center. Cephalalgia. 2022; https://doi.org/10.1177/03331024221104178.
37. Gómez-Beldarrain M, Anton-Ladislao A, Aguirre-Larracoechea U, Oroz I, García-Moncó JC. Low cognitive reserve is associated with chronic migraine with medication overuse and poor quality of life. Cephalalgia. 2014;35(8):683–91.
38. Radat F, Chanraud S, Di Scala G, Dousset V, Allard M. Psychological and neuropsychological correlates of dependence-related behaviour in medication overuse headaches: a one year follow-up study. J Headache Pain. 2013;14(1):59.
39. Dousset V, Maud M, Legoff M, Radat F, Brochet B, Dartigues JF, et al. Probable medications overuse headaches: validation of a brief easy-to-use screening tool in a headache centre. J Headache Pain. 2013;14(1):81.
40. Weaver M, Patrick DL, Markson LE, Martin D, Frederic I, Berger M. Issues in the measurement of satisfaction with treatment. Am J Manag Care. 1997;3(4):579–94.

41. Reuter U, Ehrlich M, Gendolla A, Heinze A, Klatt J, Wen S, et al. Erenumab versus topiramate for the prevention of migraine—a randomised, double-blind, active-controlled phase 4 trial. Cephalalgia. 2021;42(2):108–18.
42. López-Bravo A, Oliveros-Cid A, Sevillano-Orte L. Treatment satisfaction with calcitonin gene-related peptide monoclonal antibodies as a new patient-reported outcome measure: A real-life experience in migraine. Acta Neurologica Scandinavica. 2022;145(6):669–75.
43. Bonafede M, Cai Q, Cappell K, Kim G, Sapra SJ, Shah N, et al. Factors associated with direct health care costs among patients with migraine. J Manag Care Spec Pharm. 2017;23(11):1169–76.
44. Bigal ME, Serrano D, Buse D, Scher A, Stewart WF, Lipton RB. Acute migraine medications and evolution from episodic to chronic migraine: a longitudinal population-based study. Headache. 2008;48(8):1157–68.
45. Buse DC, Pearlman SH, Reed ML, Serrano D, Ng-Mak DS, Lipton RB. Opioid use and dependence among persons with migraine: results of the AMPP study. Headache. 2012;52(1):18–36.
46. Ashina S, Foster SA, Nicholson RA, Araujo AB, Reed ML, Shapiro RE, et al. Opioid use among people with migraine: Results of the overcome study. Headache. 2019;59:11.
47. Robbins L. Long-acting opioids for refractory chronic migraine. Pract Pain Manag. 2009;9(6)
48. Butler SF, Budman SH, Fernandez K, Jamison RN. Validation of a screener and opioid assessment measure for patients with chronic pain. Pain. 2004;112(1–2):65–75.
49. Butler SF, Budman SH, Fernandez KC, Fanciullo GJ, Jamison RN. Cross-validation of a Screener to Predict Opioid Misuse in Chronic Pain Patients (SOAPP-R). J Addict Med. 2009;3(2):66–73.
50. Aly Z, Rosen N, Evans RW. Migraine and the risk of suicide. Headache. 2016;56(4):753–61.
51. Butler SF, Budman SH, Fernandez KC, Houle B, Benoit C, Katz N, et al. Development and validation of the current opioid misuse measure. Pain. 2007;130(1-2):144–56.
52. Weaver M, Schnoll S. Addiction issues in prescribing opioids for chronic nonmalignant pain. J Addict Med. 2007;1(1):2–10.
53. Pascual J, Láinez MJ, Baos V, García ML, López-Gil A. Predictive model for the Migraine-ACT questionnaire in primary care. Curr Med Res Opin. 2007;23(12):3033–9.
54. García ML, Baos V, Láinez M, Pascual J, López-Gil A. Responsiveness of migraine-ACT and MIDAS questionnaires for assessing migraine therapy. Headache. 2008;48(9):1349–55.
55. Lipton RB, Fanning KM, Serrano D, Reed ML, Cady R, Buse DC. Ineffective acute treatment of episodic migraine is associated with new-onset chronic migraine. Neurology. 2015;84(7):688–95.
56. Davis KH, Black L, Sleath B. Validation of the Patient Perception of Migraine Questionnaire. Value Health. 2002;5(5):422–30.
57. Vollmer WM, Markson LE, O'Connor E, Sanocki LL, Fitterman L, Berger M, et al. Association of asthma control with health care utilization and quality of life. Am J Respir Crit Care Med. 1999;160(5 Pt 1):1647–52.
58. Campinha-Bacote DL, Kendle JB, Jones C, Callicoat D, Webert A, Stoukides CA, et al. Impact of a migraine management program on improving health outcomes. Dis Manag. 2005;8(6):382–91.
59. Vikelis M, Dermitzakis EV, Vlachos GS, Soldatos P, Spingos KC, Litsardopoulos P, et al. Open label prospective experience of supplementation with a fixed combination of magnesium, vitamin B2, feverfew, andrographis paniculata and coenzyme Q10 for episodic migraine prophylaxis. J Clin Med. 2020;10(1)
60. Martin ML, Patrick DL, Bushnell DM, Gandra SR, Gilchrist K. Further validation of an individualized migraine treatment satisfaction measure. Value Health. 2008;11(5):904–12. https://doi.org/10.1111/j.1524-4733.2008.00320.x. Epub 2008 May 20. PMID: 18494756.

# Chapter 11
# Other Questionnaires We Don't Want to Miss in Headache Studies

Burcu Polat, Aynur Özge, and Pınar Yalınay Dikmen

## 11.1 Introduction

Pain has idiosyncratic and intricate nature leading to strains of measurement. Yet, it is vital for physicians and researchers to apply precise tools to measure pain in evidence-based medicine. Up-to-now no valid and reliable measuring tool that objectively quantifies pain based on individual perception has been devised. For this reason, self-reporting techniques to identify the impact of pain are heavily counted on. However, it is still possible to gather the estimates of pain through several methods and scales despite existing challenges in the field. Thanks to these tools—when applied correctly—clinicians and researchers are able to demonstrate both statistically and clinically significant treatment outcomes.

Headache registries are to cover validated headache-specific surveys and patient reported outcome measures (PROMs). PROMs are applied with an aim to assess health, quality of life, or functional status associated with health care or treatment as reported by patients themselves. PROMs are of the utmost importance in headache studies as the outcomes are heavily dependent on patients' self-reports and merely subjective.

B. Polat
Department of Neurology, International School of Medicine, Istanbul Medipol University, Istanbul, Turkey
e-mail: burcupolat@medipol.edu.tr

A. Özge
Department of Neurology, Faculty of Medicine, Mersin University, Mersin, Turkey

P. Yalınay Dikmen (✉)
Department of Neurology, School of Medicine, Acıbadem University, Istanbul, Turkey
e-mail: pinar.yalinay@acibadem.edu.tr

© The Author(s), under exclusive license to Springer Nature Switzerland AG 2023
P. Yalınay Dikmen, A. Özge (eds.), *Clinical Scales for Headache Disorders*, Headache, https://doi.org/10.1007/978-3-031-25938-8_11

In this chapter, the aim is to elaborate on some of the tools addressing pain threshold, somatosensory and cognitive functions, global impression, triggers and pain acceptance and perception in patients with headache/migraine namely MIGraine Attacks-Subjective COGnitive impairments scale (Mig-SCog scale), Work Productivity and Activity Impairment Questionnaire (WPAIQ), Headache Triggers Sensitivity and Avoidance Questionnaire (HTSAQ), Patient Global Impression of Change Scale (PGICS), Patient Perception of Migraine Questionnaire—revised (PPMQ-rev), Chronic Pain Acceptance Questionnaire-8 (CPAQ-8), The Headache Acceptance Questionnaire (HAQ), The Loneliness of Migraine Scale (LMS) and Severity of Dependence Scale (SDS) and Quantitative Sensory Testing (QST).

## 11.1.1 Migraine Attacks-Subjective Cognitive Impairments Scale (Mig-SCog Scale)

Migraine is one of the major factors affecting young and dynamic population and resulting in decrease in professional competency. Furthermore, it poses significant economic lost and strains for health-care service. The impairment of cognitive function associated with migraine attacks leads to a decrease in patients' performance in work-environment, school, and in other habitats where daily activities are performed. Consequently, migraine leads to a serious clinical impact regarding migraine-related disability and the loss of workforce. Before and during migraine attacks, majority of patients complain not only about pain but also about cognitive deterioration, including increased reaction time, attention deficit, impaired concentration and visuospatial processing, episodic memory deficits, and problems with verbal learning [1–3].

However, during migraine attacks it is not convenient to apply detailed neuropsychological tests. Moreover, the available ones are either too long for daily clinical application or not precise. In 2011, Raquel Gil-Gouveia et al. developed a specific tool to measure and assess subjective cognitive symptoms during migraine attacks called Mig-SCog. It is a Likert-type scale consisting of nine items scored between 0 and 18. This scale is easy to apply, proves to be reliable, and internally consistent and has good temporal stability. The first three questions are bound up with attention/processing speed/orientation; questions 4 and 5 cover planning/attention while 6 and 7 are closely related with language; 8 and 9 refer to language: naming. Eventually, Mig-SCog highlights the domains leading to the highest number of complaints in patients during an attack, namely, executive functions (attention, planning, and orientation) and language (naming and language). A high Mig-SCog score indicates a high frequency of cognitive symptoms [4, 5]. The basic limitation of this scale is its reliance upon patients' subjective perception and sensations. It has been translated and validated into Turkish and Italian language [6, 7]. Pain and cognitive dysfunction during the migraine attack are correlated with total attack disability. The Mig-SCog scale is efficient in monitoring patients' cognitive complaints and assessing response to pharmacotherapy, particularly during attacks. Cognitive performance is to be conceived as a secondary endpoint in clinical trials of drugs for acute migraine treatment. A report has been published on the clinical experience in an Italian real-world setting using Erenumab in patients with chronic migraine who previously experienced unsuccessful preventive treatments—as assessed by Mig-SCog—did not show statistically significant improvement after either the third or sixth administrations. Although symptoms such as pain severity, pain-related quality of life, and allodynia improved with Erenumab treatment, no change was found in attack-related cognitive impairment [8]. Mig-SCog seems to be a promising tool for future studies and should be studied more.

### 11.1.2   Work Productivity and Activity Impairment Questionnaire (WPAI)

Headache and migraine are major reasons of "lost" days due to absenteeism [9]. Furthermore, not only absenteeism but also presenteeism because of migraine is a leading cause of workplace productivity loss. In 2016, migraine was graded as the second highest reason of disability at aged 15–49 years by the Global Burden of Disease [10]. This information has a great impotence for the public health perspective, and it is known that headache disorders have socioeconomic consequences. However, it seems to the neglected-health problem. There is a paucity of evidence on the impact of migraine and other headache disorders in addition to the cost and loss of capability in the workplace [11]. The extent to which the headache related loss of professional efficiency could be evaluated on the WPAI questionnaire, which is an instrument to measure impairments in both paid work and unpaid work. Reilly et al. developed this questionnaire to measure the effect of general health and symptom severity on work productivity and regular activities. Unlike general health or disease-specific measures, this questionnaire assessed function-related endpoints to allow a measure of the economic impact of relative differences in either the safety or efficacy of therapeutic interventions. The WPAI was created as a patient-reported quantitative assessment of the amount of absenteeism, presenteeism and daily activity impairment attributable to general health (WPAI: GH) or a specific health problem (WPAI: SHP) [9, 10]

The WPAI yields four types of scores: (1) Absenteeism (work time missed), (2) Presenteeism (impairment at work/reduced on-the-job effectiveness), (3) Work productivity loss (overall work impairment/absenteeism plus presenteeism) and (4) Activity Impairment (http://www.reillyassociates.net/Index.html). The WPAI: GH and the WPAI: SHP were devised simultaneously and had the same template. The subject is instructed to respond with reference to general health status in the GH version, while the subject responds with reference to a specified health problem, disease, or condition in the SHP version. WPAI questionnaire elicited the numbers of days and hours missed from work, days and hours worked, days during which performance was low and the extent to which the individual was limited at work (work impairment) during the past 7 days. The extent of professional inefficiency and impairment, attributable to ill-health and the symptom or problem specified by the respondent was elicited. Scores were measured as percentages of scheduled work hours performed and productivity observed at work on workdays [12]. Blumenfeld et al. assessed headache impact, depression, functioning and daily living, activity, and work productivity to measure the effectiveness of onabotulinumtoxinA compared with topiramate in people with chronic migraine. They administered this test on day 1 and at weeks 12, 24, and 36. The patients who switched to onabotulinumtoxinA also completed the instrument at week 48. Changes from baseline at week 36 favored onabotulinumtoxinA treatment compared with topiramate across domains on the WPAI:SHP. In Work Productivity Loss domain, there was a significant difference in reduction in impairment score from baseline among patients treated with onabotulinumtoxinA compared with topiramate. In the Activity Impairment domain, a significantly larger change from baseline was also observed among patients treated with onabotulinumtoxinA [13]. This scale can be used in clinical practice or drug studies, especially in terms of monitoring efficiency at work for patients with migraine.

### 11.1.3  *The Headache Triggers Sensitivity and Avoidance Questionnaire (HTSAQ)*

Avoiding triggering factors of headache is the first advice provided to patients by clinicians. Indeed, studies have shown that short exposure to a headache trigger causes increased sensitivity and prolonged exposure results in diminish sensitivity. The HTSAQ lists 24 of the most commonly reported triggers for headaches and using a 5-point Likert-scale assesses respondents' sensitivity to these triggers, as well as their avoidance of these triggers [14]. Indeed, the main limitation of HTSAQ is that the questionnaire relies on self-report data and hence is subject to all the issues associated with such data. To exemplify, "are respondents aware of how sensitive they are to triggers compared with others", or "how sensitive are they nowadays compared with the past?". Furthermore, "can headache sufferers even accurately identify what the triggering factors of their headaches are?" [15]. This questionnaire is made up 24 of the most frequently mentioned triggers (stress, odors, lack of sleep, etc.) as well as two open questions for individual triggers that can be added. The triggers are each rated on four scales. For each trigger, it is recorded on a 5-point Likert scale: (1) how often the respondent experiences headaches because of the trigger (scale Triggers); (2) how sensitive the respondent is to the trigger compared with other people (scale S(O)); (3) how sensitive the respondent is to the trigger compared with the time of least sensitivity (scale S(T)); and (4) how hard the respondent tries to avoid the trigger (scale Avoidance). For the Triggers scale there are response options ranging from 1 = "Never" to 5 = "Always", for the scale S(O) from 1 = "Not at all sensitive" to 5 = "Very highly sensitive", for the scale S(T) from 1 = "Same" to 5 = "Very much more sensitive", and for the scale Avoidance from 1 = "Do not try at all to avoid" to 5 = "Try to avoid at all costs" The questionnaire is rather long with at least 88 items to answer. Therefore, this questionnaire needs to be simplified [16].

HTSAQ-SF is a short version of this questionnaire. Both the long and short forms of the questionnaire appear to be reliable and have valid measures. The development of the short form of the questionnaire simplifies the use of the HTSAQ in clinical practice [16]. The advantages of this questionnaire involve individual and unique therapy provision and prognosis. Future academic studies are expected to address whether the use of the HTSAQ remains to be efficient compared to other diagnostic instruments (e.g., questionnaires to measure pain anxiety and pain acceptance).

### 11.1.4 *Patient Global Impression of Change Scale (PGIC)*

Another self-reporting tool PGIC projects a patient's belief about the efficacy of treatment. PGIC is an integrated measure of drug tolerability and efficacy, measuring the patient's view of improvement or decline in clinical status after the drug exposure. PGIC is a 7-point scale reflecting a patient's rating of overall improvement. Patients rate their change as "very much improved," "much improved," "minimally improved," "no change," "minimally worse," "much worse," or "very much worse." PGIC is frequently applied in clinical trials regarding monoclonal antibodies and is correlated with significant treatment improvement. PGIC scale mainly measures change in clinical status. The PROM is related to the patient's perspective as it is likely to be the most essential factor to consider when evaluating the impact of treatment. In fact, the patients' perception of a treatment has been associated with treatment adherence. Thus, asking the patients to rate their change in their migraine when taking a preventive treatment using the PGIC could be a valuable instrument since it is easy to apply and not so time-consuming. For this reason, it is to be introduced in clinical practice [17, 18]. The clinical relevance of the PGIC is currently guaranteed by allowing patients to specify the factors they reckon important for their health status. Additionally, due to the large placebo effect often seen in migraine research, the "improved" group in the PGIC is defined using the two highest PGIC response categories (i.e., "very much improved" and "much improved"), which is compared to a "not improved" group combining five responses from "minimally improved" to "very much worse."

### 11.1.5  Patient Perception of Migraine Questionnaire-Revised (PPMQ-R)

Patients' perceptions towards to therapy plays an important role for clinicians' treatment decisions and patients' compliances. The Patient Perception of Migraine Questionnaire is one of the few published questionnaires assessing patient satisfaction with acute migraine treatment during the first 4 weeks. The first validation study of this questionnaire was published in 2002. Authors recommended some minor modifications to the questionnaire including addition of one item (side effects) and deletion of several redundant items [19]. PPMQ-Revised version consists of 32 items, of which 29 are core items (items included in the subscales) and 3 are global items (individual items that measure overall satisfaction with medication effectiveness, side effects, and general treatment). The core instrument consists of 19 items evaluating satisfaction with medication covering attributes on efficacy (11 items), function (4 items), ease of use (2 items), and cost (2 items), with response options ranging from "very satisfied" to "very dissatisfied" on a 7-point Likert scale. The three global items regarding overall satisfaction with medication effectiveness, side effects, and general treatment, using the same 7-point Likert scale. The ten items evaluating how bothered the respondents were by selected medication-related side effects, with response options ranging from "not at all" to "extremely" on a 5-point Likert scale. The different response scales selected to be consistent with the content of the questions. The PPMQ-R items, excluding the global items, measure satisfaction with efficacy, function, ease of use, cost and tolerability of side effects (i.e. Efficacy, Functionality, Ease of Use, Cost and Tolerability scales). The psychometric properties of the PPMQ-R were previously evaluated in an outpatient population of adult patients from 50 primary care and neurology specialty clinics across the United States of America (n = 200). This study has displayed that the tool has good reliability and validity characteristics in both single-attack and multiple attack evaluations. In addition, the PPMQ-R was responsive to changes in clinical status of migraine attacks [20, 21]. PPMQ-R should consider as a reliable PROM in future clinical research and routine practice settings as measures of migraine-treatment response.

### 11.1.6  Chronic Pain Acceptance Questionnaire (CPAQ-8)

Between 2 and 4% of the general population suffer from chronic headache. Headache disorders are likely to affect deeply an individual's functional ability and quality of life. Affecting primarily young adults, the personal and economic burden of headache are substantial and comparable to other chronic conditions such as congestive heart failure, hypertension, or diabetes [22]. Acceptance is a potentially valuable concept in contemporary theories of how patients react and adapt to chronic pain. Pain acceptance is conceived as an essential step for pain management and its higher acceptance is correlated with less depression and anxiety [23]. Recent research suggests that pain-related acceptance leads to enhanced emotional and physical functioning in patients with chronic pain above and beyond the influence of depression, pain intensity, and coping. There are questionnaires for measurement of acceptance. They have been used in headache studies. In these studies, acceptance was measured using the CPAQ. Chronic pain acceptance, from a contextual perspective, includes experiencing ongoing pain without any effort to avoid, reduce, or otherwise control it. Two related behavioral processes have been identified including taking part in everyday activities of value to the individual in the presence of pain and staying away from the struggle to limit contact with pain. CPAQ was originally developed by Geisser in an unpublished doctoral dissertation and subsequently revised by McCracken, Vowles and Eccleston. Four factors that were labeled in the study are as follows: (1) taking part in normal life activities; (2) believing that controlling thoughts controls pain; (3) acknowledging the chronicity of pain; and (4) necessity to avoid or control pain. The second factor was later determined to be divergent from the overall construct as it was poorly correlated with the other factors and the total score [23, 24].

CPAQ is a 20-item self-report tool that assesses acceptance and experiential avoidance and is specific to pain experience. In line with the notion that acceptance of pain involves both getting involved in essential activities despite pain and being willing to bear pain, the measure consists of 2 subscale scores: activity engagement and pain willingness. Factor analytic studies have verified a 2-factor structure supporting these subscales. Higher scores for each of the scales is indicative of greater acceptance of chronic pain. CPAQ displays good internal consistency across a variety of pain syndromes of migraine, and predictive validity (correlations with pain intensity and interference [24]. It has been translated and validated into German, Spanish, Chinese, Swedish, Persian, Turkish, Italian, Norwegian and Korean.

Treatment providers and researchers often explore shorter and more time efficient means of collecting information from patient reports. Hence, a shorter version of the CPAQ has recently been developed. The result, an 8-item version of the instrument (CPAQ-8) tested in different contexts, appears to have good psychometric properties and the same 2-factor structure as the original [25]. CPAQ-8 may be a valuable clinical tool in reflecting changes in pain acceptance during treatment, which, in turn, is likely to be a fruitful strategy for treatment development.

### *11.1.7   The Headache Acceptance Questionnaire (HAQ)*

Headache acceptance is a distinct psychological construct that is meaningfully affiliated with variables of prognostic importance. Acceptance is likely to be a crucial factor lessening the painful experience of emotional functions. It is also a predictor of patient performance in the future. Strategies based on the acceptance implies on the reduction of pain symptoms and enhancing the quality of life along with pain. The main theoretical construct of acceptance is based on behavioral treatments such as acceptance and commitment therapy and psychological flexibility. It means the ability to take effective action in line with personal values despite the presence of pain [26].

Despite its verified importance as a psychological process of headache disorders, tools to assess acceptance of headache are still lacking. The 20-item CPAQ is the most applied measure of pain acceptance. However, it was devised and validated among individuals with chronic musculoskeletal pain. Therefore, it fails to reveal unique aspects of headache diseases, in particular responses to interictal periods in the absence of pain or avoidance of potential attack trigger. Furthermore, its length restricts routine use in medical settings. Therefore, it is vital to formulate and validate a brief measure that assesses acceptance of head pain. The six-item HAQ evaluates acceptance of headache and has been proved to be efficient in providing promising initial psychometric characteristics incorporating convergent validity with measures of disability and related constructs, as well as divergent validity with a measure of social desirability, and the ability to distinguish between diagnostic groups. Acceptance of headache is conceived to be a vital factor in clinical contexts as it is likely to be a standpoint to lessen headache disease-related disability and shall be the core point in treatment outcomes and mechanisms of change [27]. Among a broad sample of adults with a variety of headache presentations, headache acceptance scores had strong inverse associations with headache-related disability and fear of pain paving way to the initial studies on general pain acceptance among individuals with migraine [28, 29]. Individuals with tension type headache reported greater headache acceptance than those with more severe and disabling forms of headache (e.g. migraine, cluster, post-traumatic) This further supporting the construct validity of the scale.

### 11.1.8   The Loneliness of Migraine Scale (LMS)

Loneliness can be defined as a discrepancy between desired and actual social contacts. Broadening the sense of the term, four additional dimensions of loneliness, depending on whether it is literal or figurative, sought actively, or forced upon a person are aimed to be distinguished. "Literal loneliness" can be defined as absence of other people; "figurative loneliness", on the other hand, refers to a feeling or expectation of lacking social support and being on one's own. Neumeier et al in their study assumed that these four dimensions to be relevant for migraine. At first, it is common that patients actively isolate themselves during a migraine attack. Then, passive loneliness can occur between the episodes, and might result from avoidance behavior and anxiety. Further, literally being lonely and feeling lonely stem from very different emotional states. As previous studies showed that the ictal burden is only one aspect of the disease burden—albeit an important one— some authors have claimed that loneliness might be a crucial factor triggering the interictal burden. Moreover, loneliness is likely underreported possibly because it grows slowly over time and might remain unnoticed by patients, their surroundings, and treating physicians over long periods. Perhaps, shame might also prevent patients from naming such feelings. Neumeier et al developed and validated the LMS in 2022. The LMS is a reliable and valid questionnaire measuring the loneliness of migraine patients. Feelings of loneliness are common and correlated highly with migraine days, anxiety, and depression [30]. The LMS' development and validation study included slightly more men than women, and more women than men are affected by migraine in the general population, their sample might not be representative. Moreover, the number of participants was limited. Additionally, there are some methodological inadequacies of this scale. Thus, further studies are required to confirm the psychometric characteristics of the loneliness on migraine scale.

### 11.1.9 *Severity of Dependence Scale (SDS)*

Migraine attacks recur episodically in majority of cases; however, a small percentage of patients becomes chronic. It is well-known that medication overuse headache (MOH) is highly common in patients with chronic migraine. The presence of medication overuse and addiction-like behaviors affect a usage of both acute and prophylactic drugs and follow-up strategies of patients with chronic migraine. Even simple analgesics are not "safe" in the treatment of chronic headache. In fact, every drug requires awareness of the possibility of drug abuse and addiction. Therefore, MOH should always be kept in mind in the management of migraine treatment.

SDS is widely applied to evaluate the severity of dependence among substance users. SDS is a five-item questionnaire measuring psychological components of dependence. The SDS consists of five questions rated with a score of 0–3. The scale has been proved to be valid and reliable in the general population, across substances and settings [31]. The higher scores indicate a higher degree of dependence. SDS has high capability to confirm and rule out the presence of medication misuse and dependence. The strength of this scale is that it is simple, easily applicable and time efficient. SDS is conceived to be a promising screening tool for dependency-like behaviors in patients with chronic migraine and MOH [32, 33]. SDS has also been applied in the cases of MOH, where it was shown to be a predictor of MOH in samples of primary chronic headache patients from Norwegian population [33]. Bottiroli et al. assessed dependence from medications in a large sample of Italian chronic migraine and MOH [32].

However, there is a lot to be scientifically disclosed in headache field. Knowledge on burden of medication misuse or dependency-like behaviors of headache patients is limited and healthcare systems is insufficient for enabling general practitioners and public health officials to develop and implement evidence-based strategies for early detection, prevention, and treatment. Those patients bearing the risk of dependency-like behaviors require a referral to level 3. SDS could assist future research in predicting risk factors as well as consequences of medication overusing and dependency-like behaviors in headache patients.

## *11.1.10  Quantitative Sensory Testing (QST)*

Migraine is a complex, basically inherited variable disorder of brain function. Undoubtedly there is a lot to be revealed on how we comprehend migraine. It is most likely that many of the ideas surrounding its pathophysiology are relevant, from a genetic predisposition to brain hyperexcitability, to peripheral and central sensitization, and brain stem and hypothalamic dysfunction [34]. Migraine attacks occur due to a disorder of brain sensory processing that itself likely cycles, influenced by genetics and the environmental factors. Quantitative sensory testing (QST), exercised with especially in clinical therapeutic trials, measures sensory thresholds for pain, touch, vibration, and hot and cold temperature sensations. There are devices varying from hand-held tools to sophisticated computerized equipment with complicated testing algorithms, standardization of stimulation and recording procedures. Through these tests, specific fiber functions can be assessed: $A\delta$-fibers with cold, cold-pain, and mechanical pain detection thresholds; C-fibers with heat and heat-pain detection thresholds; and large fiber ($A\alpha\beta$-) functions with vibration detection thresholds and mechanical detection thresholds to von Frey hairs. Elevated sensory thresholds correlate with sensory loss; lowered thresholds occur in allodynia and hyperalgesia. Certain QST findings may relate to specific pathophysiologic mechanisms associated with neuropathic pain: heat hyperalgesia to peripheral sensitization and static mechanical hyperalgesia or dynamic mechanical allodynia to central sensitization [35]. QST can be used in conditions with chronic pain. Migraine is one of them and QST has been used to evaluate and quantify altered somatosensory functions in patients with migraine. Although QST has been extensively applied in patients with migraine for more than 50 years, there is still lack of standardization. Different laboratories apply different stimulation modalities (heat, cold, pressure, etc.), measures (thresholds, suprathreshold stimuli, and pain modulation), and locations. In the meta-analysis of QST studies on migraine, Nahman-Averbuch et al. concluded that the alterations in nociceptive processing of patients with migraine may be modality, measure, and location specific [36]. As for the shortcomings of QST are that it has never been used to differentiate between neuropathic and nonneuropathic pains, and QST abnormalities occur in nonneuropathic pain conditions. Abnormal findings are not specific for peripheral nerve dysfunction, whereas central nervous system disorders shall also affect sensory thresholds. The most significant bottleneck is that QST is a subjective psychophysical test entirely dependent upon patient motivation, alertness, and concentration. Patients can deliberately perform poorly, and even when not doing so, there are large intra- and interindividual variations [35]. Given the complex psychosocial and psychological components associated with individual pain thresholds, the diagnosis of pain syndromes is not to be reached solely based on QST. There is inadequate evidence to support the use of QST in monitoring heat pain thresholds in response to therapeutic agents. Although there is limited Class II evidence to suggest that QST may be useful in demonstrating altered thresholds for pain perception in patients with various pain syndromes, the sensitivity and specificity of QST in the diagnosis of such disorders are unclear (Level U recommendation) [37]. This does not indicate that other QST protocols will not differentiate patients with migraine from healthy controls but suggests that a larger sample size is to be required to find out this difference. Another possibility is that this test is relevant to the mechanisms of migraine and could be used as predictors for the migraine development or treatment success. Szikszay et al. published their findings' and strongly suggested that patients with migraine have a disrupted offset analgesia (OA) which distinguishes migraine from healthy controls. What is more astonishing is the fact that from this study OA in migraine is somatotopically disrupted with intact pain modulation outside the trigeminal V1 system, whereas the magnitude of the OA does not seem to be different in all body sites checked. The question comes forth whether migraine specific needs to be addressed in future research [38]. Burstein et al. were the first to demonstrate the development of an allodynia with a typical spatial and temporal distribution during migraine attacks [39]. The application of QST in research has displayed that the presence of cutaneous allodynia, a clinical manifestation of central sensitization, can be detrimental to the success of migraine therapy with different drugs [40].

## 11.2 Conclusion

In busy clinical setting, healthcare professionals may often be an unaware of degree and extent of functional impairment caused by migraine. Clinicians might miss opportunity to provide effective acute treatment and preventive pharmacological and biobehavioral interventions in that case. It means that ictal and inter ictal burden of migraine may increase for a patient in time. Clinical scales and PROMs give chance to clinicians further comprehensive evaluation of patients' status besides ictal burden of migraine. Researchers in headache medicine have an opportunity to evaluate not only a personal but also social and economic burden of migraine by means of some of these instruments. In this chapter, we introduced to readers a recently created and less widely applied scales and PROMs. We intend to increase clinicians' awareness about these instruments and to help to publicize them. Accurate assessments of patients with migraine have a critical importance for creating the most appropriate treatment strategy for individuals. Therefore, clinical scales and PROMs are assessment tools that assist to clinicians and researchers for measuring individual needs of patients with headache and help to formulating the best treatment choices for them.

## References


1. Mulder EJ, Linssen WH, Passchier J, Orlebeke JF, de Geus EJ. Interictal and postictal cognitive changes in migraine. Cephalalgia. 1999;19:557–65.
2. Vuralli D, Ayata C, Bolay H. Cognitive dysfunction and migraine. J Headache Pain. 2018;19:109.

3. Gil-Gouveia R, Martins IP. Clinical description of attack-related cognitive symptoms in migraine: A systematic review. Cephalalgia. 2018;38:1335–50.

4. Gil-Gouveia R, Oliveira AG, Martins IP. A subjective cognitive impairment scale for migraine attacks. The MIG-SCOG: development and validation. Cephalalgia. 2011;31:984–91.

5. Gil-Gouveia R, Oliveira AG, Martins IP. The impact of cognitive symptoms on migraine attack-related disability. Cephalalgia. 2016;36:422–30.

6. Polat B, Özge A, Yılmaz NH, Taşdelen B, Düz ÖA, Kılıç S, et al. Validity and reliability of the Turkish version of the Mig-Scog scale in migraine patients. Neurol Sci Neurophysiol. 2020;37:29–35.

7. Russo A, Silvestro M, Garramone F, Tessitore A, Cropano M, Scotto di Clemente F, et al. A subjective cognitive impairments scale for migraine attacks: validation of the Italian version of the MIG-SCOG. Neurol Sci. 2020;41:1139–43.

8. Russo A, Silvestro M, Scotto di Clemente F, Trojsi F, Bisecco A, Bonavita S, et al. Multidimensional assessment of the effects of erenumab in chronic migraine patients with previous unsuccessful preventive treatments: a comprehensive real-world experience. J Headache Pain. 2020;21:69.

9. Baigi K, Stewart WF. Headache and migraine: a leading cause of absenteeism. Handb Clin Neurol. 2015;131:447–63.

10. Vos T, Abajobir AA, Abate KH, Abbafati C, Abbas KM, Abd-Allah F, et al. Global, regional, and national incidence, prevalence, and years lived with disability for 328 diseases and injuries for 195 countries, 1990-2016: a systematic analysis for the Global Burden of Disease Study 2016. Lancet. 2017;390:1211–59.

11. Shimizu T, Sakai F, Miyake H, Sone T, Sato M, Tanabe S, et al. Disability, quality of life, productivity impairment and employer costs of migraine in the workplace. J Headache Pain. 2021;22:29.

12. Reilly MC, Zbrozek AS, Dukes EM. The validity and reproducibility of a work productivity and activity impairment instrument. Pharmacoeconomics. 1993;4:353–65.

13. Blumenfeld AM, Patel AT, Turner IM, Mullin KB, Manack Adams A, Rothrock JF. Patient-reported outcomes from a 1-year, real-world, head-to-head comparison of onabotulinumtoxinA and topiramate for headache prevention in adults with chronic migraine. J Prim Care Community Health. 2020;11:2150132720959936.

14. Sullivan DP, Martin PR. Sleep and headaches: Relationships between migraine and non-migraine headaches and sleep duration, sleep quality, chronotype, and obstructive sleep apnea risk. Aust J Psychol. 2017;69:210–7.

15. Kubik SU, Martin PR. The Headache Triggers Sensitivity and Avoidance Questionnaire: establishing the psychometric properties of the questionnaire. Headache. 2017;57:236–54.

16. Caroli A, Klan T, Gaul C, Kubik SU, Martin PR, Witthöft M. Types of triggers in migraine—factor structure of the Headache Triggers Sensitivity and Avoidance Questionnaire and Development of a New Short Form (HTSAQ-SF). Headache. 2020;60:1920–9.

17. Alpuente A, Gallardo VJ, Caronna E, Torres-Ferrus M, Pozo-Rosich P. In search of a gold standard patient-reported outcome measure to use in the evaluation and treatment-decision making in migraine prevention. A real-world evidence study. J Headache Pain. 2021;22:151.

18. William G. Clinical global impressions. In: ECDEU assessment manual for psychopharmacology—revised. Rockville: National Institute of Mental Health; 1976. p. 218–22.

19. Davis KH, Black L, Sleath B. Validation of the Patient Perception of Migraine Questionnaire. Value Health. 2002;5:422–30.

20. Revicki DA, Kimel M, Beusterien K, Kwong JW, Varner JA, Ames MH, et al. Validation of the revised Patient Perception of Migraine Questionnaire: measuring satisfaction with acute migraine treatment. Headache. 2006;46:240–52.

21. Kimel M, Hsieh R, McCormack J, Burch SP, Revicki DA. Validation of the revised Patient Perception of Migraine Questionnaire (PPMQ-R): measuring satisfaction with acute migraine treatment in clinical trials. Cephalalgia. 2008;28:510–23.

22. Haywood KL, Mars TS, Potter R, Patel S, Matharu M, Underwood M. Assessing the impact of headaches and the outcomes of treatment: A systematic review of patient-reported outcome measures (PROMs). Cephalalgia. 2018;38:1374–86.
23. Seng EK, Kuka AJ, Mayson SJ, Smitherman TA, Buse DC. Acceptance, psychiatric symptoms, and migraine disability: an observational study in a headache center. Headache. 2018;58:859–72.
24. McCracken LM, Vowles KE, Eccleston C. Acceptance of chronic pain: component analysis and a revised assessment method. Pain. 2004;107:159–66.
25. Fish RA, McGuire B, Hogan M, Morrison TG, Stewart I. Validation of the chronic pain acceptance questionnaire (CPAQ) in an Internet sample and development and preliminary validation of the CPAQ-8. Pain. 2010;149:435–43.
26. Gharaee-Ardakani Sh AP, Eydi-Baygi M, Zafarizade A, Tork M. Effect of acceptance and commitment therapy on the acceptance of pain and psychological inflexibility among women with chronic headache. J Res Health. 2017;7:729–35.
27. Hamer JD, Sackey ET, Maack DJ, Smitherman TA. Development of a measure to assess acceptance of headache: The Headache Acceptance Questionnaire (HAQ). Cephalalgia. 2020;40:797–807.
28. Chiririos C, O'Brien WH. Acceptance, appraisals, and coping in relation to migraine headache: an evaluation of interrelationships using daily diary methods. J Behav Med. 2011;34:307–20.
29. Foote HW, Hamer JD, Roland MM, Landy SR, Smitherman TA. Psychological flexibility in migraine: A study of pain acceptance and values-based action. Cephalalgia. 2016;36:317–24.
30. Neumeier M, Pohl H, Gantenbein A. The loneliness of migraine scale: a development and validation study. Clin Transl Neurosci. 2022;6
31. Gossop M, Darke S, Griffiths P, Hando J, Powis B, Hall W, et al. The Severity of Dependence Scale (SDS): psychometric properties of the SDS in English and Australian samples of heroin, cocaine and amphetamine users. Addiction (Abingdon, England). 1995;90:607–14.
32. Bottiroli S, Galli F, Ballante E, Pazzi S, Sances G, Guaschino E, et al. Validity of the Severity of Dependence Scale for detecting dependence behaviors in chronic migraine with medication overuse. Cephalalgia. 2022;42:209–17.
33. Grande RB, Aaseth K, Saltyte Benth J, Gulbrandsen P, Russell MB, Lundqvist C. The Severity of Dependence Scale detects people with medication overuse: the Akershus study of chronic headache. J Neurol Neurosurg Psychiatry. 2009;80:784–9.
34. Goadsby PJ, Holland PR, Martins-Oliveira M, Hoffmann J, Schankin C, Akerman S. Pathophysiology of migraine: a disorder of sensory processing. Physiol Rev. 2017;97:553–622.
35. Smith HS. Current therapy in pain. Philadelphia: Saunders/Elsevier; 2009.
36. Nahman-Averbuch H, Shefi T, Schneider VJ 2nd, Li D, Ding L, King CD, et al. Quantitative sensory testing in patients with migraine: a systematic review and meta-analysis. Pain. 2018;159:1202–23.
37. Shy ME, Frohman EM, So YT, Arezzo JC, Cornblath DR, Giuliani MJ, et al. Quantitative sensory testing. Neurology. 2003;60:898–904.
38. Szikszay TM, Adamczyk WM, Carvalho GF, May A, Luedtke K. Offset analgesia: somatotopic endogenous pain modulation in migraine. Pain. 2020;161:557–64.
39. Burstein R, Cutrer MF, Yarnitsky D. The development of cutaneous allodynia during a migraine attack clinical evidence for the sequential recruitment of spinal and supraspinal nociceptive neurons in migraine. Brain. 2000;123:1703–9.
40. Landy S, Rice K, Lobo B. Central sensitization and cutaneous allodynia in migraine: implications for treatment. CNS Drugs. 2004;18:337–42.

# Chapter 12
# Clinical Scales for Special Groups

Daniel N. Lax and Andrew D. Hershey

## 12.1   Introduction

Pain and emotion are subjective continuous variables and thus can be challenging to measure. This is especially true for younger patients and research subjects who may not be able to use scales previously developed for adults. Therefore, pain and psychiatric scales should be validated in the population of interest prior to their use for clinical and research purposes. This applies to scales already validated in adults as well as new scales developed especially for the youngest of our population. Similarly, parent and caregiver perception tools developed for younger children or those with developmental differences should be validated against the self-perception tools available. As children and adolescents live very different lives from adults, school-specific tools have been developed as well. Clinical and research guidelines include use of scales and tools for youth in research and clinical practice. In this chapter we review the most commonly used and recommended scales and tools for use in children and adolescents for both these purposes. This includes scales for pain severity, disability, psychiatric comorbidities, and a school-based tool.

D. N. Lax (✉)
Division of Neurology, Cincinnati Children's Hospital Medical Center, Cincinnati, OH, USA

Department of Neurology, Montefiore Medical Center, Albert Einstein College of Medicine, Bronx, NY, USA
e-mail: dalax@montefiore.org

A. D. Hershey
Division of Neurology, Cincinnati Children's Hospital Medical Center, Cincinnati, OH, USA

Department of Pediatrics, University of Cincinnati College of Medicine, Cincinnati, OH, USA
e-mail: Andrew.Hershey@cchmc.org

© The Author(s), under exclusive license to Springer Nature Switzerland AG 2023
P. Yalınay Dikmen, A. Özge (eds.), *Clinical Scales for Headache Disorders*, Headache, https://doi.org/10.1007/978-3-031-25938-8_12

## 12.2  Pain Severity Scales

An integral part of the headache history is pain severity as diagnostic criteria for migraine include moderate to severe pain [1]. Additionally, severity of attacks may help guide treatment. While adults typically do not have trouble rating pain on various numerical scales, such scales may be developmentally inappropriate for younger children. To address this, a number of visual aids have been developed. These aids can be used both clinically in acute (emergency department, inpatient) and chronic (outpatient clinic) settings and as primary or secondary endpoints for research purposes [2].

Broadly, pain scales in children include self-report measures and parent or caregiver perception, with the former serving as the preferred primary measure when possible [3]. Self-report tools include visual analog scales (VAS), numeric rating scales (NRS), color analog scales (CAS), pieces of hurt (POH) tool and faces scales. While more detailed scales may deliver a greater likelihood of statistically significant changes in severity for research purposes, the abstract construct of all but the latter two limit their use in younger children. However, the POH tool has not been validated for recurrent or chronic pain in children and relies on obtaining and maintaining individual chips requiring cleaning between patients or subjects. As numeric and analog scales are discussed in the adult chapters and faces scales are generally preferred over the others for younger children, we will focus on the latter here [4, 5].

In the 1980s Wong and Baker noted that younger children had considerable difficulty with scales using numbers or words, and when they were able to use adult scales, they were not believed. Instead, they asked children to retrospectively draw their various levels of pain in six empty circles. Thus, the Wong-Baker FACES® Pain Rating Scale was developed. In its current form, it consists of six images of faces beginning with a smiley face indicating no pain on the left with increasingly uncomfortable-appearing faces to the right with an image of a face crying with tears as the greatest severity (see Fig. 12.1). It is psychometrically sound and has been validated in adults and children as young as 3 years old. The leading critique of this scale relates to the images at either extreme. The smile face can bias pain scores toward more severe levels, while the tears may bias older children toward less severe

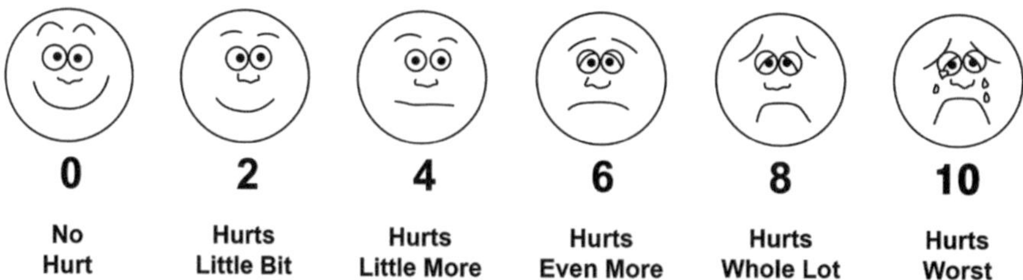


**Fig. 12.1** Wong-Baker FACES® Pain Rating Scale. © 1983 Wong-Baker FACES® Foundation. www.WongBakerFACES.org. Used with permission. Originally published in *Whaley & Wong's Nursing Care of Infants and Children.* © Elsevier Inc.

levels. Additionally, these anchors may represent measures of affect, a confounder limiting its use in clinical trials [4]. Despite these issues, the Wong-Baker scale is preferred over other faces scales by children and caregivers in acute and chronic causes of pain [6].

The Faces Pain Scale-Revised (FPS-R), based off the original Faces Pain Scale first published in the 1990s, has been validated for use in children older than 4 years old and in both acute and chronic pain-related conditions. It consists of six images of faces similar to the Wong-Baker scale but the no pain indicator consists of a neutral expression and most severe pain does not include tears. The avoidance of smiling and crying anchors is a potential benefit over the Wong–Baker scale and it is therefore more widely used for research purposes. It appears to be the most psychometrically sound instrument for younger children, though less pre-ferred by older children and adolescents when compared to alternative faces scales and other tools [4].

The Oucher tool consists of photographs of children with corresponding numeri-cal values displayed vertically increasing in pain severity and grade from bottom up. It has adequate psychometric properties and has been validated in many forms dif-fering in their photographs of male and female children of various ethnicities. The anchor is non-smiling but the lack of gender and ethnic neutrality and cost of color printing make its clinical and research use more challenging [4]. All three of these faces scales have been translated into dozens of languages.


## 12.3  Disability Scales

The majority of migraine-related disability scales used for adults have not been vali-dated in youth, and children are not just little adults. The daily lives of children and adolescents differ considerably from those of adults, so the assessment of migraine effects on their lives should be correspondingly distinct. For example, the Migraine Disability Assessment (MIDAS) discussed in chapter, is heavily weighted toward work, household chores and leisure with less accounting for partial days of work missed, whereas partial days of school missed are an important and possibly more common factor clinically relevant for children with migraine [7]. Similarly, while an adult's job responsibilities should theoretically end at work, a child's education continues with homework. As practice guidelines for both acute and preventive management of migraine in children include an assessment of disability [8, 9], an appropriate evaluation tool is crucial. Further, guidelines for clinical trials in chil-dren and adolescents with migraine recommend a validated assessment of disability as an outcome measure [2], specifically citing the Pediatric Migraine Disability Assessment (PedMIDAS).

The PedMIDAS is a six-question self-assessment of disability validated for use in children and adolescents [7] and has been translated into multiple languages. Similar to the MIDAS, patients are asked to quantify number of days unable to per-form certain functions during the previous 3 months. One main addition is the assessment of partial school days missed. In addition, instead of assessing reduction of household responsibility productivity and complete loss of leisure activities, PedMIDAS measures decreased function performing homework/chores AND leisure activities. In essence, PedMIDAS asks three questions about school-related disability and three questions about non-school related disability. It has demonstrated reliability and validity and is easy to use even without direct physician contact. One limitation described is a relative underestimate of disability on non-school days since a single school day can theoretically score 3 points (missed full day of school, missed homework, missed sports) whereas a non-school day maxes out at 2 points (missed homework, missed sports) [10].

The Functional Disability Inventory (FDI)-Child and Adolescent Form was similarly developed based on its adult version [11]. It replaces verbiage relevant to adults with developmentally appropriate items applicable to the status of younger children. It consists of 15 questions assessing function in home, school, social and recreational settings using a 5-point Likert scale. Validity and consistency were supported through multiple studies of youth with both "organic" and "functional" abdominal pain and remains one of the most widely used measures of disability in those with chronic pain, headache, hematologic, oncologic and gastrointestinal disorders [12]. Validity was based on correlation with school absenteeism and there was also a strong correlation with parent form of the FDI. Clinically useful reference points for interpretation of FDI scores were developed later but it had already been in use for a number of headache-related studies. The National Institute of Neurological Disorders and Stroke (NINDS) common data elements (CDE) lists PedMIDAS as "Supplemental-Highly Recommended" and FDI as "Supplemental" for functional outcomes for clinical trials in pediatrics [13].

The Pediatric Quality of Life Inventory (PedsQL) is a validated 4-min, 23-item tool covering physical, emotional, social and school domains. The self-report can be completed by youth ages 8 years and older with interviewer-administered questionnaire for ages 5–7. A proxy report is available for ages 2 and up and there is even an infant version for ages 1–24 months through caregiver reports. There is evidence for its reliability in a sample of 2–18-year-olds with migraine [14] and has been validated for use in children with recurrent headache [15] and in youth with traumatic brain injury.

## 12.4 Psychiatric Comorbidity Assessment Scales

The observation that children with migraine commonly suffer from comorbid psychological disorders was first published in the 1950s [16]. Since then, much effort has been devoted to measuring the association of anxiety and depression with headache disorders. Specifically, children with migraine and/or tension type headache have been found to show greater psychopathological symptoms than healthy controls. Depression and anxiety seem to predict migraine persistence and higher depression score predicts greater migraine-related disability at follow-up. Guidelines for prevention therapies recommend screening children and adolescents with migraine for mood and anxiety disorders because of this risk of headache persistence [8] and some medications used for migraine prevention in children can have negative mood effects. Similarly, guidelines for clinical trials of preventive treatment of migraine in children and adolescents recommend recording depression and anxiety levels at time of randomization and at the end of treatment period [2]. A number of depression and anxiety scales are available for use in youth with migraine (see Table 12.1).

The original full version Patient Health Questionnaire for Adolescents (PHQ-A) was the first validated tool assessing anxiety, mood, eating and substance use disorders in adolescents. In lieu of this long multi-domain instrument, brief disorder-specific versions have since been tested in adolescents, including the 9-item PHQ-9 and 2-item PHQ-2 which consists of the first 2 items of the PHQ-9 [17]. Since the dimensional algorithm of PHQ-9 was superior to PHQ-2, a suggested method of screening uses a low threshold ($\geq 2$ points) on the PHQ-2 for greater sensitivity to warrant further screening with PHQ-9 which has greater specificity and includes

**Table 12.1** Psychiatric comorbidity assessment scales

| Name of tool | Pediatric age range | Psychiatric domain | Application to headache |
|---|---|---|---|
| PHQ-9 modified for teens | 11–17 years | Depression | Listed in IHS guidelines for preventive trials in children and adolescents [2]<br>Listed as "Supplemental Highly Recommended" for emotional status outcomes in pediatrics by NINDS CDE [13] |
| PHQ-2 | 12–17 years | | |
| GAD-7 | 11–17 years | Anxiety | Listed in IHS guidelines for preventive trials in children and adolescents [2]<br>Listed as "Supplemental Highly Recommended" for emotional status outcomes in pediatrics by NINDS CDE [13] |
| CDI-2 | 7–17 years | Depression | Listed as "Pediatric Recommendation" for emotional status outcomes by NINDS CDE [13] |
| HADS | 12–17 years | Anxiety and Depression | Listed in IHS guidelines for preventive trials in children and adolescents [2]<br>Listed as "Supplemental" for emotional status outcomes by NINDS CDE [13] |
| BDI-II | 13–17 years | Depression | Listed in IHS guidelines for preventive trials in children and adolescents [2]<br>Listed as "Supplemental" for emotional status outcomes by NINDS CDE [13] |
| STAI-Y | 14–17 years | Anxiety | STAI-Y listed in IHS guidelines for preventive trials in children and adolescents [2]<br>STAI listed as "Supplemental" for emotional status outcomes by NINDS CDE [13] |
| STAI-C | 8–13 years | | |
| PROMIS | 8–17 years | Multiple domains | PROMIS Anxiety and Depression Scales listed as "Pediatric Recommendation" for patient reported outcomes by NINDS CDE [13] |

assessment of suicidality. Modified versions of the PHQ-9 for adolescent/teen use are available. A potential confounder of these tools is that many of the symptoms queried in the PHQ-9 may also be symptoms of migraine attacks, such as poor appetite and difficulty with sleep, etc. [18]. In addition, the Diagnostic and Statistical Manual of Mental Disorders fifth edition (DSM-5) allows for irritable mood to replace depressed mood in children and adolescents, something not reflected in the PHQ-9.

The Pediatric Anxiety Rating Scale (PARS) has been validated for assessing and trending anxiety symptoms in children 6–17 years old [19] but is limited by the 30-min administration time. The Generalized Anxiety Disorder 7-item Scale (GAD-7) is a 2-min self-assessment tool which correlates well with PARS for detecting moderate to severe generalized anxiety disorder in adolescents [20]. Similar to PHQ-9, some symptoms assessed by GAD-7 overlap with symptoms inherent to migraine. Both PHQ-9 and GAD-7 have been validated for use in migraine, though not in the pediatric and younger adolescent age groups. Both the PHQ-9 and GAD-7 are listed in NINDS CDE as "Supplemental Highly Recommended" outcome measures of emotional status, though not specifically for the pediatric population. PHQ and GAD tools are available online at no cost in many languages (https://www.phqscreeners.com/select-screener) and PHQ-A and GAD-7 are specifically recommended in the International Headache Society (HIS) guidelines for preventive treatment trials in children and adolescents [2].

The Children Depression Inventory-2 (CDI-2) is listed as "Pediatric Recommendation" for emotional status outcomes by NINDS CDE [13]. The full version is comprised of three forms: self-report, teacher report and parent report with an estimated length of 10–15 min. The short version is estimated to take 5 min and is specifically for screening purposes. The full versions assess emotional and functional problems with subcategories of mood/physical symptoms and self-esteem for the former and ineffectiveness and interpersonal problems for the latter [21]. Both versions are based on the last 2 weeks of information so it may be used as a measure of treatment efficacy both clinically and experimentally in relatively short periods. It has been validated for use in youth aged 7–17 years.

The CDI-2 was based off the Beck Depression Inventory (BDI) with modifications for developmental appropriateness in younger children. The second edition (BDI-II) is also included in guidelines for clinical trials in children and adolescents [2]. This tool uses a 4-point rating scale of 21 items based on a 2-week timeframe, a modification of the 1-week timeframe of the original version to better comply with DSM-IV criteria. It has been validated in those aged 13–80 years [22]. Both CDI-2 and BDI-II can be purchased from http://pearsonassess.com/.

The Hospital Anxiety and Depression Scale (HADS) uses seven items each to assess anxiety and depression on a 4-point Likert scale and has been validated for use in adolescents [23]. A lower cutoff for increased sensitivity is recommended in adolescents compared to adults. A unique attribute of the HADS is that it does not include somatic symptoms and may therefore be more suitable for screening adolescents with physical illness or headaches causing physical symptom which overlap with depression and anxiety. However, since DSM criteria for anxiety and depression include somatic symptoms, their omission from HADS may increase the rate of false negatives. This omission and overrepresentation of anhedonia symptoms has generated considerable criticism. A meta-analysis found little evidence of HADS superiority to other screening tools in detecting specific mental health disorders in those with physical illness [24].

The State-Trait Anxiety Inventory (STAI) is a 20-item self-report tool which has been used in pediatric pain research with Form-Y for older children (STAI-Y) and Form-C for younger children (STAI-C). The inclusion of both state, or current level of anxiety as well as trait, or generalized long-term anxiety, is considered a unique benefit of this tool. In addition, the value of a parent version has been demonstrated in conjunction with self-report inventories [25]. Despite the frequent use of these tools, there is limited evidence for their validity in youth with chronic disease.

The Patient-Reported Outcomes Measurement Information System (PROMIS) pediatric anxiety and depressive symptoms instruments are validated tools for use in youth aged 8–17 years [26] with proxy tools for ages 5–17 years. The items in these scales are part of a large National Institutes of Health funded collaborative for the development of computerized self-reported outcomes within a wide variety of diseases. PROMIS Anxiety and Depression Scales are listed as "Pediatric Recommendation" for patient reported outcomes by NINDS CDE [13], has been used in studies of headache-related disability in teens [27] and has evidence for validity in pediatric traumatic brain injury [28]. The scales assess experiences within the past week and both the full and short versions are available for free (https://www.healthmeasures.net/explore-measurement-systems/promis).

## 12.5  School Based Tool

Not infrequently, the first contact of a child with recurrent headaches will be their school nurse. School nurses are in the unique position of witnessing the child during a typical school day which is a common setting for headache attacks. The Pediatric and Adolescent Migraine Screen (PAMS) tool was developed with this in mind. It is an ultra-brief 3-item screening tool for detecting migraine in school-age youth and is available at no cost [29]. Once migraine is suspected, school nurses could recommend further evaluation for diagnosis and treatment thus avoiding unnecessary delays to care.

## 12.6  Conclusion

Children are not just little adults, so they should not be treated as such. When available, tools validated for use in youth should be utilized based on the national and international guidelines discussed throughout this chapter. When planning clinical encounters or research endeavors, these guidelines should be reviewed and implemented for best clinical practice and to ensure standardization of clinical trials in children and adolescents with migraine.

# References


1. Headache Classification Committee of the International Headache Society (IHS). The International Classification of Headache Disorders, 3rd edition. Cephalalgia. 2018;38(1):1–211. https://doi.org/10.1177/0333102417738202.
2. Abu-Arafeh I, Hershey AD, Diener H-C, Tassorelli C. Guidelines of the International Headache Society for controlled trials of preventive treatment of migraine in children and adolescents, 1st edition. Cephalalgia. 2019;39(7):803–16. https://doi.org/10.1177/0333102419842188.
3. Zhou H, Roberts P, Horgan L. Association between self-report pain ratings of child and parent, child and nurse and parent and nurse dyads: meta-analysis. J Adv Nurs. 2008;63(4):334–42. https://doi.org/10.1111/j.1365-2648.2008.04694.x.
4. Tomlinson D, von Baeyer CL, Stinson JN, Sung L. A systematic review of faces scales for the self-report of pain intensity in children. Pediatrics. 2010;126(5):e1168–e98. https://doi.org/10.1542/peds.2010-1609.
5. Stinson JN, Kavanagh T, Yamada J, Gill N, Stevens B. Systematic review of the psychometric properties, interpretability and feasibility of self-report pain intensity measures for use in clinical trials in children and adolescents. Pain. 2006;125(1):143–57. https://doi.org/10.1016/j.pain.2006.05.006.
6. Chambers CT, Giesbrecht K, Craig KD, Bennett SM, Huntsman E. A comparison of faces scales for the measurement of pediatric pain: children's and parents' ratings. Pain. 1999;83(1):25–35. https://doi.org/10.1016/s0304-3959(99)00086-x.
7. Hershey AD, Powers SW, Vockell AL, LeCates S, Kabbouche MA, Maynard MK. PedMIDAS: development of a questionnaire to assess disability of migraines in children. Neurology. 2001;57(11):2034–9. https://doi.org/10.1212/wnl.57.11.2034.
8. Oskoui M, Pringsheim T, Billinghurst L, Potrebic S, Gersz EM, Gloss D, et al. Practice guideline update summary: Pharmacologic treatment for pediatric migraine prevention: Report of the Guideline Development, Dissemination, and Implementation Subcommittee of the American Academy of Neurology and the American Headache Society. Headache. 2019;59(8):1144–57. https://doi.org/10.1111/head.13625.
9. Oskoui M, Pringsheim T, Holler-Managan Y, Potrebic S, Billinghurst L, Gloss D, et al. Practice guideline update summary: Acute treatment of migraine in children and adolescents. Neurology. 2019;93(11):487. https://doi.org/10.1212/WNL.0000000000008095.
10. Heyer GL, Merison K, Rose SC, Perkins SQ, Lee JM, Stewart WC. PedMIDAS-based scoring underestimates migraine disability on non-school days. Headache. 2014;54(6):1048–53. https://doi.org/10.1111/head.12327.
11. Walker LS, Greene JW. The functional disability inventory: measuring a neglected dimension of child health status. J Pediatr Psychol. 1991;16(1):39–58. https://doi.org/10.1093/jpepsy/16.1.39.
12. Palermo TM, Long AC, Lewandowski AS, Drotar D, Quittner AL, Walker LS. Evidence-based assessment of health-related quality of life and functional impairment in pediatric psychology. J Pediatr Psychol. 2008;33(9):983–98. https://doi.org/10.1093/jpepsy/jsn038.
13. https://www.commondataelements.ninds.nih.gov/sites/nindscde/files/Doc/Headache/Headache_CDE_Highlight_Summary.pdf. Accessed April 21, 2022.
14. Powers SW, Patton SR, Hommel KA, Hershey AD. Quality of life in paediatric migraine: Characterization of age-related effects using PedsQL 4.0. Cephalalgia. 2004;24(2):120–7. https://doi.org/10.1111/j.1468-2982.2004.00652.x.
15. Connelly M, Rapoff MA. Assessing health-related quality of life in children with recurrent headache: reliability and validity of the PedsQL™ 4.0 in a pediatric headache sample. J Pediatr Psychol. 2006;31(7):698–702. https://doi.org/10.1093/jpepsy/jsj063.
16. Vahlquist B. Migraine in children. Int Arch Allergy Immunol. 1955;7(4–6):348–55. https://doi.org/10.1159/000228238.

17. Allgaier AK, Pietsch K, Frühe B, Sigl-Glöckner J, Schulte-Körne G. Screening for depression in adolescents: validity of the patient health questionnaire in pediatric care. Depress Anxiety. 2012;29(10):906–13. https://doi.org/10.1002/da.21971.
18. Qubty W, Gelfand AA. Psychological and behavioral issues in the management of migraine in children and adolescents. Curr Pain Headache Rep. 2016;20(12):69. https://doi.org/10.1007/s11916-016-0597-1.
19. The Research Units On Pediatric Psychopharmacology Anxiety Study Group. The Pediatric Anxiety Rating Scale (PARS): development and psychometric properties. J Am Acad Child Adolesc Psychiatry. 2002;41(9):1061–9. https://doi.org/10.1097/00004583-200209000-00006.
20. Mossman SA, Luft MJ, Schroeder HK, Varney ST, Fleck DE, Barzman DH, et al. The Generalized Anxiety Disorder 7-item scale in adolescents with generalized anxiety disorder: Signal detection and validation. Ann Clin psychiatry. 2017;29(4):227–34A.
21. Bae Y. Test Review: Children's Depression Inventory 2 (CDI 2). J Psychoeduc Assess. 2012;30(3):304–8. https://doi.org/10.1177/0734282911426407.
22. Osman A, Kopper BA, Barrios F, Gutierrez PM, Bagge CL. Reliability and validity of the Beck depression inventory—II with adolescent psychiatric inpatients. Psychol Assess. 2004;16(2):120–32. https://doi.org/10.1037/1040-3590.16.2.120.
23. White D, Leach C, Sims R, Atkinson M, Cottrell D. Validation of the Hospital Anxiety and Depression Scale for use with adolescents. Br J Psychiatry. 1999;175:452–4. https://doi.org/10.1192/bjp.175.5.452.
24. Brennan C, Worrall-Davies A, McMillan D, Gilbody S, House A. The Hospital Anxiety and Depression Scale: a diagnostic meta-analysis of case-finding ability. J Psychosom Res. 2010;69(4):371–8. https://doi.org/10.1016/j.jpsychores.2010.04.006.
25. Shain LM, Pao M, Tipton MV, Bedoya SZ, Kang SJ, Horowitz LM, et al. Comparing parent and child self-report measures of the state-trait anxiety inventory in children and adolescents with a chronic health condition. J Clin Psychol Med Settings. 2020;27(1):173–81. https://doi.org/10.1007/s10880-019-09631-5.
26. Bevans KB, Gardner W, Pajer KA, Becker B, Carle A, Tucker CA, et al. Psychometric evaluation of the PROMIS® pediatric psychological and physical stress experiences measures. J Pediatr Psychol. 2018;43(6):678–92. https://doi.org/10.1093/jpepsy/jsy010.
27. Kemper KJ, Heyer G, Pakalnis A, Binkley PF. What factors contribute to headache-related disability in teens? Pediatr Neurol. 2016;56:48–54. https://doi.org/10.1016/j.pediatrneurol.2015.10.024.
28. Bertisch H, Rivara FP, Kisala PA, Wang J, Yeates KO, Durbin D, et al. Psychometric evaluation of the pediatric and parent-proxy patient-reported outcomes measurement information system and the neurology and traumatic brain injury quality of life measurement item banks in pediatric traumatic brain injury. Qual Life Res. 2017;26(7):1887–99. https://doi.org/10.1007/s11136-017-1524-6.
29. https://www.cincinnatichildrens.org/service/h/headache-center/pams (2007). Accessed April 21, 2022.

# Appendix

## Development and Validation of the Headache Needs Assessment (HANA) Survey

**Appendix.—Headache Needs Assessment (HANA) Questionnaire**

*We are interested in knowing how you feel about having migraine headaches and the problems caused by your headaches in usual daily activities. This information will help us to understand the problems you face related to having frequent and severe migraine headaches. Please answer questions A and B for each problem listed (1–7) describing how migraine headaches affected your life in the past 4 weeks.*

| Problem area: | Question A | Question B |
|---|---|---|
| | How often has this problem occurred? 1 = never, 2 = rarely, 3 = sometimes, 4 = often, 5 = all the time | How much has this problem bothered you? 1 = not at all, 2 = a little, 3 = some, 4 = a lot, 5 = a great deal |
| In the **past month**, . . . | | |
| Problem 1. I have felt **anxious or worried** (tense, wound-up, frightened) about having another severe headache. | | |
| Problem 2. I have felt **depressed, discouraged** about my headaches. | | |
| Problem 3. I have felt that I am not in **control** of myself because of my headaches. | | |
| Problem 4. I have had less **energy**; I am more **tired** than I should have been because of my headaches. | | |
| Problem 5. I **functioned** and **worked** (attention, concentration, etc.) at a lower level than I should have because of my headaches. | | |
| Problem 6. I have felt that my **family and social activities** were limited because of my headaches. | | |
| Problem 7. I have felt that my **life centered or revolved** around my headaches. | | |

*Thank you for taking time to describe living with your headaches.*



JA Cramer, SD Silberstein, P Winner. Development and validation of the Headache Needs Assessment (HANA) survey. Headache 2001;41(4):402-9. **DOI:** https://doi.org/10.1046/j.1526-4610.2001.111006402.x

© The Editor(s) (if applicable) and The Author(s), under exclusive license to Springer Nature Switzerland AG 2023
P. Yalınay Dikmen, A. Özge (eds.), *Clinical Scales for Headache Disorders*, Headache, https://doi.org/10.1007/978-3-031-25938-8

# The Headache Triggers Sensitivity and Avoidance Questionnaire

**APPENDIX**
**HEADACHE TRIGGERS SENSITIVITY
AND AVOIDANCE QUESTIONNAIRE
(HTSAQ)**

Headache/migraine triggers are defined as factors that alone or in combination can precipitate or aggravate headaches in susceptible individuals. Triggers can be thought of as varying in terms of "**potency**" or "**dosage,**" which may be determined by variables such as intensity of the trigger (how extreme) and duration of exposure to the trigger. For example, noise can trigger headaches, but the impact of noise is likely to be determined by how loud it is, and the length of exposure to the noise. Chocolate can trigger headaches but does it require consumption of a row of 5-6 squares (30 g), or a family block (250 g)? Lack of sleep can trigger headaches but does this mean 30-60 minutes less than usual, or the level of sleep deprivation that can arise from international plane travel (most of a night without sleep)? Headaches can be triggered by stress, but stress varies from "daily hassles" such as being caught in a traffic jam or burning the toast, to "major life events" such as being made redundant or losing a family member.

There are individual differences in "**sensitivity**" or "susceptibility" to triggers, that is, the level of potency/dosage of a trigger that is required to precipitate a headache/migraine. For example, for some individuals a very loud noise may be needed to precipitate a headache whilst for others a lower level of noise could result in a headache. Also, sensitivity to triggers can vary across time (ie, a lower or higher trigger potency/dosage may be required to precipitate a headache during different stages of life). Some individuals try to **avoid** the triggers of headaches because they do not want to experience a headache, and this tendency may be reinforced by advice from doctors or on the internet.

Listed below are the most commonly reported triggers. There are 22 triggers that potentially apply to anyone, one trigger that applies to smokers, and one trigger that applies to women only. There is space for adding up to

2 triggers that precipitate your headaches but are not on the list.

For each of the triggers listed, we would like you to answer 4 questions using the 5-point scales below the questions. The questions are about whether this potential trigger is a trigger of your headaches (question A), your sensitivity to this trigger (questions B and C), and whether you try to avoid this trigger (question D).

A. How often do you experience headaches because of this trigger?
    1. Never
    2. Rarely
    3. Sometimes
    4. Usually
    5. Always

B. How **sensitive** are you to this trigger currently compared with other people?
    1. Not at all sensitive (ie, exposure even at high intensities for prolonged periods would not precipitate a headache)
    2. Slightly sensitive
    3. Moderately sensitive
    4. Highly sensitive
    5. Very highly sensitive (ie, exposure even at very low intensities for short periods would precipitate a headache)

C. How **sensitive** are you to this trigger currently compared with how sensitive you were at the time in your life when you were least sensitive to the trigger?
    1. Same
    2. Slightly more sensitive
    3. Moderately more sensitive
    4. Much more sensitive
    5. Very much more sensitive

D. How hard do you try to **avoid** this trigger?
    1. Do not try at all
    2. Make a small effort to avoid
    3. Make a moderate effort to avoid
    4. Make a large effort to avoid
    5. Try to avoid at all costs

Please respond to each question by circling **one** number. Please remember that the 4 questions for each trigger that is, A, B, C, and D have different scales to use in responding (refer back).

| | |
|---|---|
| **1 A** How often do you experience headaches because of **stress?** | 1 2 3 4 5 |
| **1 B** How **sensitive** are you to **stress** as a trigger of headaches currently compared with other people? | 1 2 3 4 5 |
| **1 C** How **sensitive** are you to **stress** as a trigger of headaches currently compared with how sensitive you were at the time in your life when you were least sensitive to stress? | 1 2 3 4 5 |
| **1 D** How hard do you try to **avoid stress?** | 1 2 3 4 5 |
| **2 A** How often do you experience headaches because of **anxiety?** | 1 2 3 4 5 |
| **2 B** How **sensitive** are you to **anxiety** as a trigger of headaches currently compared with other people? | 1 2 3 4 5 |
| **2 C** How **sensitive** are you to **anxiety** as a trigger of headaches currently compared with how sensitive you were at the time in your life when you were least sensitive to anxiety? | 1 2 3 4 5 |
| **2 D** How hard do you try to **avoid anxiety?** | 1 2 3 4 5 |
| **3 A** How often do you experience headaches because of **anger?** | 1 2 3 4 5 |
| **3 B** How **sensitive** are you to **anger** as a trigger of headaches currently compared with other people? | 1 2 3 4 5 |
| **3 C** How **sensitive** are you to **anger** as a trigger of headaches currently compared with how sensitive you were at the time in your life when you were least sensitive to anger? | 1 2 3 4 5 |
| **3 D** How hard do you try to **avoid anger?** | 1 2 3 4 5 |
| **4 A** How often do you experience headaches because of **depression?** | 1 2 3 4 5 |
| **4 B** How **sensitive** are you to **depression** as a trigger of headaches currently compared with other people? | 1 2 3 4 5 |
| **4 C** How **sensitive** are you to **depression** as a trigger of headaches currently compared with how sensitive you were at the time in your life when you were least sensitive to depression? | 1 2 3 4 5 |
| **4 D** How hard do you try to **avoid depression?** | 1 2 3 4 5 |
| **5 A** How often do you experience headaches because of **glare?** | 1 2 3 4 5 |
| **5 B** How **sensitive** are you to **glare** as a trigger of headaches currently compared with other people? | 1 2 3 4 5 |
| **5 C** How **sensitive** are you to **glare** as a trigger of headaches currently compared with how sensitive you were at the time in your life when you were least sensitive to glare? | 1 2 3 4 5 |
| **5 D** How hard do you try to **avoid glare?** | 1 2 3 4 5 |
| **6 A** How often do you experience headaches because of **flicker?** | 1 2 3 4 5 |
| **6 B** How **sensitive** are you to **flicker** as a trigger of headaches currently compared with other people? | 1 2 3 4 5 |

**(Continued)**

**6 C** How **sensitive** are you to **flicker** as a trigger   1 2 3 4 5
of headaches currently compared with how
sensitive you were at the time in your life
when you were least sensitive to flicker?
**6 D** How hard do you try to **avoid flicker?**   1 2 3 4 5

**7 A** How often do you experience headaches   1 2 3 4 5
because of **eyestrain?**
**7 B** How **sensitive** are you to **eyestrain** as a   1 2 3 4 5
trigger of headaches currently compared with
other people?
**7 C** How **sensitive** are you to **eyestrain** as a   1 2 3 4 5
trigger of headaches currently compared with
how sensitive you were at the time in your
life when you were least sensitive to
eyestrain?
**7 D** How hard do you try to **avoid eyestrain?**   1 2 3 4 5

**8 A** How often do you experience headaches   1 2 3 4 5
because of **noise?**
**8 B** How **sensitive** are you to **noise** as a trigger   1 2 3 4 5
of headaches currently compared with other
people?
**8 C** How **sensitive** are you to **noise** as a trigger   1 2 3 4 5
of headaches currently compared with how
sensitive you were at the time in your life
when you were least sensitive to noise?
**8 D** How hard do you try to **avoid noise?**   1 2 3 4 5

**9 A** How often do you experience headaches   1 2 3 4 5
because of **odors/smells/fragrances?**
**9 B** How **sensitive** are you to **odors/smells/fra-**   1 2 3 4 5
**grances** as a trigger of headaches currently
compared with other people?
**9 C** How **sensitive** are you to **odors/smells/fra-**   1 2 3 4 5
**grances** as a trigger of headaches currently
compared with how sensitive you were at the
time in your life when you were least sensitive to odors/smells/fragrances?
**9 D** How hard do you try to **avoid odors/**   1 2 3 4 5
**smells/fragrances?**

**10 A** How often do you experience headaches   1 2 3 4 5
because of **hunger/not eating?**
**10 B** How **sensitive** are you to **hunger/not eat-**   1 2 3 4 5
**ing** as a trigger of headaches currently com-
pared with other people?
**10 C** How **sensitive** are you to **hunger/not eat-**   1 2 3 4 5
**ing** as a trigger of headaches currently com-
pared with how sensitive you were at the
time in your life when you were least sensitive to hunger/not eating?
**10 D** How hard do you try to **avoid hunger/not**   1 2 3 4 5
**eating?**

**11 A** How often do you experience headaches   1 2 3 4 5
because of **dehydration/lack of water?**
**11 B** How **sensitive** are you to **dehydration/lack**   1 2 3 4 5
**of water** as a trigger of headaches currently
compared with other people?
**11 C** How **sensitive** are you to **dehydration/lack**   1 2 3 4 5
**of water** as a trigger of headaches currently

compared with how sensitive you were at the
time in your life when you were least
sensitive to dehydration/lack of water?
**11 D** How hard do you try to **avoid**   1 2 3 4 5
**dehydration/lack of water?**

**12 A** How often do you experience   1 2 3 4 5
headaches because of **eating "headache**
**foods"?**
**12 B** How **sensitive** are you to **eating**   1 2 3 4 5
**"headache foods"** as a trigger of headaches
currently compared with other people?
**12 C** How **sensitive** are you to **eating**   1 2 3 4 5
**"headache foods"** as a trigger of headaches
currently compared with how sensitive you
were at the time in your life when you were
least sensitive to eating "headache foods"?
**12 D** How hard do you try to **avoid eating**   1 2 3 4 5
**"headache foods"?**

**13 A** How often do you experience headaches   1 2 3 4 5
because of **drinking alcohol?**
**13 B** How **sensitive** are you to **drinking alcohol**   1 2 3 4 5
as a trigger of headaches currently compared
with other people?
**13 C** How **sensitive** are you to **drinking alcohol**   1 2 3 4 5
as a trigger of headaches currently compared
with how sensitive you were at the time in
your life when you were least sensitive to
drinking alcohol?
**13 D** How hard do you try to **avoid drinking**   1 2 3 4 5
**alcohol?**

**14 A** How often do you experience headaches   1 2 3 4 5
because of **high humidity?**
**14 B** How **sensitive** are you to **high humidity**   1 2 3 4 5
as a trigger of headaches currently compared
with other people?
**14 C** How **sensitive** are you to **high humidity**   1 2 3 4 5
as a trigger of headaches currently compared
with how sensitive you were at the time in
your life when you were least sensitive to
high humidity?
**14 D** How hard do you try to **avoid high**   1 2 3 4 5
**humidity?**

**15 A** How often do you experience headaches   1 2 3 4 5
because of **high temperature?**
**15 B** How **sensitive** are you to **high tempera-**   1 2 3 4 5
**ture** as a trigger of headaches currently
compared with other people?
**15 C** How **sensitive** are you to **high tempera-**   1 2 3 4 5
**ture** as a trigger of headaches currently
compared with how sensitive you were at the
time in your life when you were least
sensitive to high temperature?
**15 D** How hard do you try to **avoid high**   1 2 3 4 5
**temperature?**

**16 A** How often do you experience headaches   1 2 3 4 5
because of **low temperature?**

1 2 3 4 5

*(Continued)*                                       *(Continued)*

**16 B** How **sensitive** are you to **low temperature** as a trigger of headaches currently compared with other people?

**16 C** How **sensitive** are you to **low temperature** 1 2 3 4 5 as a trigger of headaches currently compared with how sensitive you were at the time in your life when you were least sensitive to low temperature?

**16 D** How hard do you try to **avoid low** 1 2 3 4 5 **temperature?**

**17 A** How often do you experience headaches 1 2 3 4 5 because of a **lack of sleep?**

**17 B** How **sensitive** are you to a **lack of sleep** 1 2 3 4 5 as a trigger of headaches currently compared with other people?

**17 C** How **sensitive** are you to a **lack of sleep** 1 2 3 4 5 as a trigger of headaches currently compared with how sensitive you were at the time in your life when you were least sensitive to a lack of sleep?

**17 D** How hard do you try to **avoid** a **lack of** 1 2 3 4 5 **sleep?**

**18 A** How often do you experience headaches 1 2 3 4 5 because of an **excess of sleep?**

**18 B** How **sensitive** are you to an **excess of** 1 2 3 4 5 **sleep** as a trigger of headaches currently compared with other people?

**18 C** How **sensitive** are you to an **excess of** 1 2 3 4 5 **sleep** as a trigger of headaches currently compared with how sensitive you were at the time in your life when you were least sensitive to an excess of sleep?

**18 D** How hard do you try to **avoid** an **excess** 1 2 3 4 5 **of sleep?**

**19 A** How often do you experience headaches 1 2 3 4 5 because of **fatigue/tiredness?**

**19 B** How **sensitive** are you to **fatigue/tiredness** 1 2 3 4 5 as a trigger of headaches currently compared with other people?

**19 C** How **sensitive** are you to **fatigue/tiredness** 1 2 3 4 5 as a trigger of headaches currently compared with how sensitive you were at the time in your life when you were least sensitive to fatigue/tiredness?

**19 D** How hard do you try to **avoid fatigue/** 1 2 3 4 5 **tiredness?**

**20 A** How often do you experience headaches 1 2 3 4 5 because of **head and neck movements**?

**20 B** How **sensitive** are you to **head and neck** 1 2 3 4 5 **movements** as a trigger of headaches currently compared with other people?

**20 C** How **sensitive** are you to **head and neck** 1 2 3 4 5 **movements** as a trigger of headaches currently compared with how sensitive you were at the time in your life when you were least sensitive to head and neck movements?

**20 D** How hard do you try to **avoid head and** 1 2 3 4 5 **neck movements?**

(Continued)

**21 A** How often do you experience headaches 1 2 3 4 5 because of **coughing/sneezing?**

**21 B** How **sensitive** are you to **coughing/sneez-** 1 2 3 4 5 **ing** as a trigger of headaches currently compared with other people?

**21 C** How **sensitive** are you to **coughing/sneez-** 1 2 3 4 5 **ing** as a trigger of headaches currently compared with how sensitive you were at the time in your life when you were least sensitive to coughing/sneezing?

**21 D** How hard do you try to **avoid coughing/** 1 2 3 4 5 **sneezing?**

**22 A** How often do you experience headaches 1 2 3 4 5 because of **travel/trips/driving?**

**22 B** How **sensitive** are you to **travel/trips/driv-** 1 2 3 4 5 **ing** as a trigger of headaches currently compared with other people?

**22 C** How **sensitive** are you to **travel/trips/driv-** 1 2 3 4 5 **ing** as a trigger of headaches currently compared with how sensitive you were at the time in your life when you were least sensitive to travel/trips/driving?

**22 D** How hard do you try to **avoid travel/trips/** 1 2 3 4 5 **driving?**

If you smoke cigarettes, please respond to the questions for trigger 23, otherwise jump to the questions for trigger 24.

| **23 A** How often do you experience headaches because of **smoking cigarettes?** | 1 | 2 | 3 | 4 | 5 |
|---|---|---|---|---|---|
| **23 B** How **sensitive** are you to **smoking cigarettes** as a trigger of headaches currently compared with other people? | 1 | 2 | 3 | 4 | 5 |
| **23 C** How **sensitive** are you to **smoking cigarettes** as a trigger of headaches currently compared with how sensitive you were at the time in your life when you were least sensitive to smoking cigarettes? | 1 | 2 | 3 | 4 | 5 |
| **23 D** How hard do you try to **avoid smoking cigarettes?** | 1 | 2 | 3 | 4 | 5 |

If you are female, please respond to the questions for trigger 24, otherwise jump to the questions for triggers 25 and 26. Note, question D is not listed for trigger 24 as it is not possible to avoid.

| **24 A** How often do you experience headaches because of the **menstrual cycle?** | 1 | 2 | 3 | 4 | 5 |
|---|---|---|---|---|---|
| **24 B** How **sensitive** are you to the **menstrual cycle** as a trigger of headaches | 1 | 2 | 3 | 4 | 5 |

(Continued)

currently compared with other women?

**24 C** How **sensitive** are you to the **menstrual cycle** as a trigger of headaches currently compared with how sensitive you were at the time in your life when you were least sensitive to the **menstrual cycle**?     1  2  3  4  5

---

If there is a trigger for your headaches that does not appear in the list of 24 potential triggers above, please respond to the questions for trigger 25, and to the questions for trigger 26 if there are 2 triggers that are not listed.

---

**25 A** How often do you experience headaches because of **a factor not listed here - please specify what it is**     1  2  3  4  5

____________

**25 B** How **sensitive** are you to **the factor that you have listed** as a trigger of headaches currently compared with other people?     1  2  3  4  5

**25 C** How **sensitive** are you to **the factor that you have listed** as a trigger of headaches currently compared with how sensitive you were at the time in your life when you were least sensitive to this factor?     1  2  3  4  5

**25 D** How hard do you try to **avoid the factor that you have listed**?     1  2  3  4  5

**26 A** How often do you experience headaches because of **a second factor not listed here - please specify what it is** ____________     1  2  3  4  5

**26 B** How **sensitive** are you to **the second factor that you have listed** as a trigger of headaches currently compared with other people?     1  2  3  4  5

**26 C** How **sensitive** are you to **the second factor that you have listed** as a trigger of headaches currently compared with how sensitive you were at the time in your life when you were least sensitive to this factor?     1  2  3  4  5

**26 D** How hard do you try to **avoid the second factor that you have listed**?     1  2  3  4  5

---

# The Headache Triggers Sensitivity and Avoidance Questionnaire

Kubik SU, Martin PR. The headache triggers sensitiv- ity and avoidance questionnaire: Establishing the psychometric properties of the questionnaire. *Headache*. 2017;57:236-254.

## Brief Headache Screen

| 1 | **How often do you get severe headaches (difficult or unable to continue normal function)?** | | | | |
|---|---|---|---|---|---|
| | Daily or near daily | 3-4 days/week | 2/week - 2/month | 1/month or less | Almost never |
| 2 | **How often do you get mild or less severe headaches?** | | | | |
| | Daily or near daily | 3-4 days/week | 2/week - 2/month | 1/month or less | Almost never |
| 3 | **How often do you take pain relievers, or any medication to relieve headache symptoms?** | | | | |
| | Daily or near daily | 3-4 days/week | 2/week - 2/month | 1/month or less | Almost never |
| 4 | How often do you miss some work or leisure time because of a headache? | | | | |
| | Daily or near daily | 3-4 days/week | 2/week - 2/month | 1/month or less | Almost never |
| 5 | Are you satisfied with the current medication you use to relieve your headaches? | | | | |
| | Yes | | | No | |
| 6 | Are you taking daily prescription medicine to prevent headaches? | | | | |
| | Yes | | | No | |
| | If not, do your headaches trouble you enough to take daily preventive medication? | | | | |
| | Yes | | | No | |

The Brief Headache Screen consists of a diagnostic segment and a treatment evaluation segment. The diagnostic segment is a 3-item questionnaire (**bold**) that interrogates on frequencies of (1) severe (disabling) headache, (2) mild headache, and (3) use of symptomatic medication. **Reference:** *Maizels M, Burchette R. Rapid and sensitive paradigm for screening patients with headache in primary care settings. Headache. 2003 May;43(5):441-50. doi: 10.1046/j.1526-4610.2003.03088.x.*

# The Validity and Reproducibility of a Work Productivity and Activity Impairment Instrument

## Work Productivity and Activity Impairment Questionnaire: General Health V2.0 (WPAI:GH)

The following questions ask about the effect of your health problems on your ability to work and perform regular activities. By health problems we mean any physical or emotional problem or symptom. *Please fill in the blanks or circle a number, as indicated.*

1.  Are you currently employed (working for pay)?          ___**NO**      ____ YES
    *If NO, check "NO" and skip to question 6.*

The next questions are about the **past seven days**, not including today.

2.  During the past seven days, how many hours did you miss from work because of your health problems? *Include hours you missed on sick days, times you went in late, left early, etc., because of your health problems. Do not include time you missed to participate in this study.*

    _____HOURS

3.  During the past seven days, how many hours did you miss from work because of any other reason, such as vacation, holidays, time off to participate in this study?

    _____HOURS

4.  During the past seven days, how many hours did you actually work?

    _____HOURS *(If "0", skip to question 6.)*

**Work Productivity and Activity Impairment Questionnaire:**
**Specific Health Problem V2.0, Clinical Practice Version (WPAI:SHP, V2.0, CPV)**

The following questions ask about the effect of your PROBLEM on your ability to work and perform regular activities.  *Please fill in the blanks or circle a number, as indicated.*

1.  Are you currently employed (working for pay)?        _______ NO ___ YES
       *If NO, check "NO" and skip to question 6.*

The next questions are about the **past seven days**, not including today.

2.  During the past seven days, how many hours did you miss from work because of problems <u>associated with your PROBLEM</u>?  *Include hours you missed on sick days, times you went in late, left early, etc., because of your PROBLEM*


   _______ HOURS


3.  During the past seven days, how many hours did you miss from work because of any other reason, such as vacation, or holidays?

   _______HOURS


4.  During the past seven days, how many hours did you actually work?

   _______<u>HOURS</u>_ *(If "0", skip to question 6.)*


<u>http://www.reillyassociates.net/WPAI_General.html</u>


## Permission to Use the WPAI

Written permission is neither required nor provided to researchers using the WPAI; there are no fees to use the WPAI or the translations on this website
   **Reilly MC, Zbrozek AS, Dukes EM. The validity and reproducibility of a work productivity and activity impairment instrument. Pharmacoeconomics**, 01 Nov 1993, 4(5):353-365. DOI: https://doi.org/10.2165/00019053-199304050-0000 6 PMID: 10146874


## WPAI Scoring

<u>http://www.reillyassociates.net/WPAI_Scoring.html</u>

# Chronic Pain Acceptance Questionnaire (CPAQ)

## A.1. Chronic Pain Acceptance Questionnaire–8 (CPAQ-8)

*Directions:* Below you will find a list of statements. Please rate the truth of each statement as it applies to you by circling a number. Use the following rating scale to make your choices. For instance, if you believe a statement is "Always True", you would circle the 6 next to that statement.

| Never true | Very rarely true | Seldom true | Sometimes true | Often true | Almost always true | Always true |
|---|---|---|---|---|---|---|
| 0 | 1 | 2 | 3 | 4 | 5 | 6 |

| | | |
|---|---|---|
| 1. | I am getting on with the business of living no matter what my level of pain is | 0  1  2  3  4  5  6 |
| 2. | Keeping my pain level under control takes first priority whenever I am doing something | 0  1  2  3  4  5  6 |
| 3. | Although things have changed, I am living a normal life despite my chronic pain | 0  1  2  3  4  5  6 |
| 4. | Before I can make any serious plans, I have to get some control over my pain | 0  1  2  3  4  5  6 |
| 5. | I lead a full life even though I have chronic pain | 0  1  2  3  4  5  6 |
| 6. | When my pain increases, I can still take care of my responsibilities | 0  1  2  3  4  5  6 |
| 7. | I avoid putting myself in situations where my pain might increase | 0  1  2  3  4  5  6 |
| 8. | My worries and fears about what pain will do to me are true | 0  1  2  3  4  5  6 |

*Note.* Pain willingness scale = Items 2, 4, 7 and 8 (reverse scored), activity engagement scale = Items 1, 3, 5 and 6, total = activity engagement + pain willingness.

McCracken LM, Vowles KE, Eccleston C. Acceptance of chronic pain: component analysis and a revised assessment method. Pain. 2004;107:159–166. DOI: https://doi.org/10.1016/j.pain.2003.10.012

# The Migraine Therapy Assessment Questionnaire

**Appendix—Migraine Therapy Assessment Questionnaire (MTAQ©)**

| YES | NO | |
|-----|-----|---|
| ☐ | ☐ | Most times, I get relief from my migraine symptoms within 2 hours after I take my migraine medicine. |
| ☐ | ☐ | Most times, I can get back to what I was doing within 2 hours after I take my migraine medicine. |
| ☐ | ☐ | Most months, I get 3 or more migraines. |
| ☐ | ☐ | I take daily medicine to reduce how often I get migraines. |
| ☐ | ☐ | I know what may bring on my migraines. |
| ☐ | ☐ | Most times, I try *not* to use my migraine medicines right away. |
| ☐ | ☐ | In the past month, I missed some school, work, or other activity because of a migraine. |
| ☐ | ☐ | In the past 6 months, I had to go to an emergency or urgent care center for a migraine. |
| ☐ | ☐ | I am satisfied with my migraine treatment. |

MTAQ© is a registered trademark of and copyrighted by Merck & Co., Inc. and should not be used without permission of Merck & Co., Inc. For more information, please contact Dr. X. Henry Hu, PO Box 4, WP39-166, West Point, PA 19486 or Henry_Hu@Merck.com.

Mary Lou Chatterton PharmD, Jennifer H. Lofland PharmD, MPH, Aaron Shechter BS, Walter Scott Curtice BS, X. Henry Hu MD, MPH, PhD, Jeffrey Lenow MD, JD, Stanton N. Smullens MD, David B. Nash MD, MBA, Stephen D. Silberstein MD. Reliability and Validity of the Migraine Therapy Assessment Questionnaire. Headache 2002;42(10):1006-15. DOI: https://doi.org/10.1046/j.1526-4610.2002.02230.x

# The Development of a Survey to Measure Completeness of Response to Migraine Therapy

Please think about your overall experience with your current migraine treatment and check one box for each question below.

1a. How often does one dose of your current migraine treatment completely relieve your headache pain?

- ☐ None or almost none of the time → **SKIP TO QUESTION 2A.**
- ☐ Some of the time
- ☐ About half of the time
- ☐ Most of the time
- ☐ All or almost all of the time

1b. How quickly does your current migraine treatment completely relieve your headache pain?

- ☐ Less than 30 minutes
- ☐ 30 minutes to 1 hour
- ☐ 1 hour to 2 hours
- ☐ More than 2 hours

2a. When you have a migraine, how often do you experience neck/shoulder pain?

- ☐ None or almost none of the time → **SKIP TO QUESTION 3A.**
- ☐ Some of the time
- ☐ About half of the time
- ☐ Most of the time
- ☐ All or almost all of the time

2b. How often does one dose of your current migraine treatment completely relieve your

neck/shoulder pain when you experience neck/shoulder pain with a migraine?

☐   None or almost none of the time → **SKIP TO QUESTION 3A.**

☐   Some of the time

☐   About half of the time

☐   Most of the time

☐   All or almost all of the time

2c. How quickly does your current migraine treatment completely relieve your neck/shoulder pain?

☐   Less than 30 minutes

☐   30 minutes to 1 hour

☐   1 hour to 2 hours

☐   More than 2 hours

3a. When you have a migraine, how often do you experience nausea?

☐   None or almost none of the time → **SKIP TO QUESTION 4A.**

☐   Some of the time

☐   About half of the time

☐   Most of the time

☐   All or almost all of the time

3b. How often does one dose of your current migraine treatment completely relieve your nausea

when you experience nausea with a migraine?

☐   None or almost none of the time → **SKIP TO QUESTION 4A.**

☐   Some of the time

☐   About half of the time

☐   Most of the time

☐   All or almost all of the time

3c. How quickly does your current migraine treatment completely relieve your nausea?

    ☐ Less than 30 minutes

    ☐ 30 minutes to 1 hour

    ☐ 1 hour to 2 hours

    ☐ More than 2 hours

4a. When you have a migraine, how often do you experience sensitivity to light?

    ☐ None or almost none of the time. → **<u>SKIP TO QUESTION 5A.</u>**

    ☐ Some of the time

    ☐ About half of the time

    ☐ Most of the time

    ☐ All or almost all of the time

4b. How often does one dose of your current migraine treatment completely relieve your sensitivity to light when you experience sensitivity to light with a migraine?

    ☐ None or almost none of the time → **<u>SKIP TO QUESTION 5A.</u>**

    ☐ Some of the time

    ☐ About half of the time

    ☐ Most of the time

    ☐ All or almost all of the time

4c. How quickly does your current migraine treatment completely relieve your sensitivity to light?

    ☐ Less than 30 minutes

    ☐ 30 minutes to 1 hour

    ☐ 1 hour to 2 hours

    ☐ More than 2 hours

5a. When you have a migraine, how often do you experience sensitivity to sound?

☐   None or almost none of the time → **SKIP TO QUESTION 6A.**

☐   Some of the time

☐   About half of the time

☐   Most of the time

☐   All or almost all of the time

5b. How often does one dose of your current migraine treatment completely relieve your sensitivity to sound when you experience sensitivity to sound with a migraine?

☐   None or almost none of the time → **SKIP TO QUESTION 6A.**

☐   Some of the time

☐   About half of the time

☐   Most of the time

☐   All or almost all of the time

5c. How quickly does your current migraine treatment completely relieve your sensitivity to sound?

☐   Less than 30 minutes

☐   30 minutes to 1 hour

☐   1 hour to 2 hours

☐   More than 2 hours

6a. When you have a migraine, how often do you experience irritability or moodiness?

☐   None or almost none of the time → **SKIP TO QUESTION 7.**

☐   Some of the time

☐   About half of the time

☐   Most of the time

☐   All or almost all of the time

6b. How often does one dose of your current migraine treatment completely relieve your irritability or moodiness when you experience irritability or moodiness with a migraine?

    ☐ None or almost none of the time → **<u>SKIP TO QUESTION 7.</u>**

    ☐ Some of the time

    ☐ About half of the time

    ☐ Most of the time

    ☐ All or almost all of the time

6c. How quickly does your current migraine treatment completely relieve your irritability or moodiness?

    ☐ Less than 30 minutes

    ☐ 30 minutes to 1 hour

    ☐ 1 hour to 2 hours

    ☐ More than 2 hours

7. How quickly are you able to concentrate or think clearly after taking your current migraine treatment?

    ☐ Less than 30 minutes

    ☐ 30 minutes to 1 hour

    ☐ 1 hour to 2 hours

    ☐ 2 hours to 4 hours

    ☐ More than 4 hours

8. How quickly are you able to resume your normal activities after taking your current migraine treatment?

☐ Less than 30 minutes

☐ 30 minutes to 1 hour

☐ 1 hour to 2 hours

☐ 2 hours to 4 hours

☐ More than 4 hours

9. How quickly do you get back to <u>functioning</u> normally (100%) after taking your current migraine treatment?

☐ Less than 30 minutes

☐ 30 minutes to 1 hour

☐ 1 hour to 2 hours

☐ 2 hours to 4 hours

☐ More than 4 hours

10. How quickly do you get back to <u>feeling</u> completely normal (100%) after taking your current migraine treatment?

☐ Less than 30 minutes

☐ 30 minutes to 1 hour

☐ 1 hour to 2 hours

☐ 2 hours to 4 hours

☐ More than 4 hours

11. Using your current migraine treatment, how often do your migraines come back within 24 hours?

    ☐ None or almost none of the time

    ☐ Some of the time

    ☐ About half of the time

    ☐ Most of the time

    ☐ All or almost all of the time

12. When you get a migraine, how confident are you that one dose of your current treatment will completely relieve your migraine within 2 hours?

    ☐ Not at all confident

    ☐ Somewhat confident

    ☐ Very confident

13. Once your migraine is relieved by your current treatment, how confident are you that your migraine will not come back within 24 hours?

    ☐ Not at all confident

    ☐ Somewhat confident

    ☐ Very confident

To answer the following questions, please compare the study medication with the migraine medication that you used most often prior to starting this study (i.e., your previous medication).

1.  Which medication provided more <u>complete</u> migraine relief?

    ☐   My previous medication worked a lot better.

    ☐   My previous medication worked a little better.

    ☐   Both medications worked the same.

    ☐   The study medication worked a little better.

    ☐   The study medication worked a lot better.

2.  Which medication provided <u>quicker</u> migraine relief?

    ☐   My previous medication worked a lot quicker.

    ☐   My previous medication worked a little quicker.

    ☐   Both medications worked the same.

    ☐   The study medication worked a little quicker.

    ☐   The study medication worked a lot quicker.

3.  Which medication provided <u>longer-lasting</u> migraine relief (i.e., prevented symptoms from coming back within 24 hours)?

    ☐   My previous medication worked a lot longer.

    ☐   My previous medication worked a little longer.

    ☐   Both medications worked the same.

    ☐   The study medication worked a little longer.

    ☐   The study medication worked a lot longer.

4.  Which medication allowed you to function more normally after treatment?

☐  I functioned a lot more normally after taking my previous medication.

☐  I functioned a little more normally after taking my previous medication.

☐  Both medications worked the same.

☐  I functioned a little more normally after taking my study medication.

☐  I functioned a lot more normally after taking my study medication.

5.  With which medication did you experience less fatigue (e.g., felt less tired) after treatment?

☐  I experienced a lot less fatigue with my previous medication.

☐  I experienced a little less fatigue with my previous medication.

☐  Both medications worked the same.

☐  I experienced a little less fatigue with my study medication.

☐  I experienced a lot less fatigue with my study medication.

6.  With which medication did you feel more confident that one dose would completely relieve your migraine within 2 hours?

☐  I felt a lot more confident with my previous medication.

☐  I felt a little more confident with my previous medication.

☐  I felt equally confident with both medications.

☐  I felt a little more confident with the study medication.

☐  I felt a lot more confident with the study medication.

7. With which medication did you feel more confident that your migraine would not come back within

   24 hours?

   ☐   I felt a lot more confident with my previous medication.

   ☐   I felt a little more confident with my previous medication.

   ☐   I felt equally confident with both medications.

   ☐   I felt a little more confident with the study medication.

   ☐   I felt a lot more confident with the study medication.

8. Overall, with which medication were you more satisfied?

   ☐   I was a lot more satisfied with my previous medication.

   ☐   I was a little more satisfied with my previous medication.

   ☐   I was equally satisfied with both medications.

   ☐   I was a little more satisfied with the study medication.

   ☐   I was a lot more satisfied with the study medication.

# The Development of a Survey to Measure Completeness of Response to Migraine Therapy

CD Coon, SE Fehnel, KH Davis, MC Runken, ME Beach, RK Cady. The development of a survey to measure completeness of response to migraine therapy. Headache 2012;52(4):550-72. **DOI:** https://doi.org/10.1111/j.1526-4610.2012.02099.x

# The Hospital Anxiety and Depression Scale

**Hospital Anxiety and Depression Scale (HADS)**

**Tick the box beside the reply that is closest to how you have been feeling in the past week.
Don't take too long over you replies: your immediate is best.**

| D | A | | D | A | |
|---|---|---|---|---|---|
| | | **I feel tense or 'wound up':** | | | **I feel as if I am slowed down:** |
| | 3 | Most of the time | 3 | | Nearly all the time |
| | 2 | A lot of the time | 2 | | Very often |
| | 1 | From time to time, occasionally | 1 | | Sometimes |
| | 0 | Not at all | 0 | | Not at all |
| | | | | | |
| | | **I still enjoy the things I used to enjoy:** | | | **I get a sort of frightened feeling like 'butterflies' in the stomach:** |
| 0 | | Definitely as much | | 0 | Not at all |
| 1 | | Not quite so much | | 1 | Occasionally |
| 2 | | Only a little | | 2 | Quite Often |
| 3 | | Hardly at all | | 3 | Very Often |
| | | | | | |
| | | **I get a sort of frightened feeling as if something awful is about to happen:** | | | **I have lost interest in my appearance:** |
| | 3 | Very definitely and quite badly | 3 | | Definitely |
| | 2 | Yes, but not too badly | 2 | | I don't take as much care as I should |
| | 1 | A little, but it doesn't worry me | 1 | | I may not take quite as much care |
| | 0 | Not at all | 0 | | I take just as much care as ever |
| | | | | | |
| | | **I can laugh and see the funny side of things:** | | | **I feel restless as I have to be on the move:** |
| 0 | | As much as I always could | | 3 | Very much indeed |
| 1 | | Not quite so much now | | 2 | Quite a lot |
| 2 | | Definitely not so much now | | 1 | Not very much |
| 3 | | Not at all | | 0 | Not at all |
| | | **Worrying thoughts go through my mind:** | | | **I look forward with enjoyment to things:** |
| | 3 | A great deal of the time | 0 | | As much as I ever did |
| | 2 | A lot of the time | 1 | | Rather less than I used to |
| | 1 | From time to time, but not too often | 2 | | Definitely less than I used to |
| | 0 | Only occasionally | 3 | | Hardly at all |
| | | | | | |
| | | **I feel cheerful:** | | | **I get sudden feelings of panic:** |
| 3 | | Not at all | | 3 | Very often indeed |
| 2 | | Not often | | 2 | Quite often |
| 1 | | Sometimes | | 1 | Not very often |
| 0 | | Most of the time | | 0 | Not at all |
| | | | | | |
| | | **I can sit at ease and feel relaxed:** | | | **I can enjoy a good book or radio or TV program:** |
| | 0 | Definitely | 0 | | Often |
| | 1 | Usually | 1 | | Sometimes |
| | 2 | Not Often | 2 | | Not often |
| | 3 | Not at all | 3 | | Very seldom |

Please check you have answered all the questions

<u>Scoring:</u>
Total score: Depression (D) _____________          Anxiety (A) _______________
0-7      = Normal
8-10    = Borderline abnormal (borderline case)
11-21  = Abnormal (case)

Zigmond, A. S., & Snaith, R.P. (1983). The Hospital Anxiety And Depression Scale, Acta Psychiatrica Scandinavica, 67, 361-370. **https://doi.org/10.1111/j.1600-0447.1983.tb09716.x**

# EuroQoL Quality of Life Scale (EQ-5D)

## Health Questionnaire (EQ-5D-5L)

Under each heading, please tick the ONE box that best describes your health TODAY.

**MOBILITY**
- ☐₁ I have no problems in walking about
- ☐₂ I have slight problems in walking about
- ☐₃ I have moderate problems in walking about
- ☐₄ I have severe problems in walking about
- ☐₅ I am unable to walk about

**SELF-CARE**
- ☐₁ I have no problems washing or dressing myself
- ☐₂ I have slight problems washing or dressing myself
- ☐₃ I have moderate problems washing or dressing myself
- ☐₄ I have severe problems washing or dressing myself
- ☐₅ I am unable to wash or dress myself

**USUAL ACTIVITIES** *(e.g. work, study, housework, family or leisure activities)*
- ☐₁ I have no problems doing my usual activities
- ☐₂ I have slight problems doing my usual activities
- ☐₃ I have moderate problems doing my usual activities
- ☐₄ I have severe problems doing my usual activities
- ☐₅ I am unable to do my usual activities

**PAIN / DISCOMFORT**
- ☐₁ I have no pain or discomfort
- ☐₂ I have slight pain or discomfort
- ☐₃ I have moderate pain or discomfort
- ☐₄ I have severe pain or discomfort
- ☐₅ I have extreme pain or discomfort

**ANXIETY / DEPRESSION**
- ☐₁ I am not anxious or depressed
- ☐₂ I am slightly anxious or depressed
- ☐₃ I am moderately anxious or depressed
- ☐₄ I am severely anxious or depressed
- ☐₅ I am extremely anxious or depressed

- We would like to know how good or bad your health is **TODAY**.

- This scale is numbered from 0 to 100.

- 100 means the <u>best</u> health you can imagine.
  0 means the <u>worst</u> health you can imagine.

- Mark an X on the scale to indicate how your health is **TODAY**

- Now, please write the number you marked on the scale in the

  below.

YOUR HEALTH TODAY =

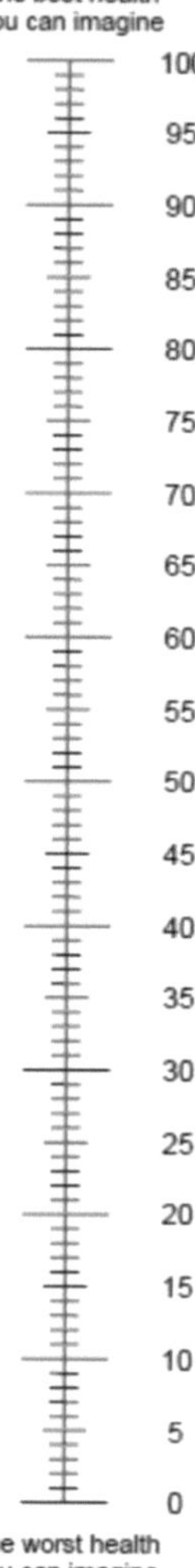




The EuroQual Group. EuroQoL - a new facility for the measurement of health-related quality of life. Health Policy 1990;16:199-208. DOI: https://doi.org/10.1016/0168-8510(90)90421-9

# Short Form 36 (SF-36)

## SF-36 QUESTIONNAIRE

**Name:**_____________________    **Ref. Dr:**________________    **Date:** _______

**ID#:** ______________    **Age:** _______    **Gender: M / F**

Please answer the 36 questions of the **Health Survey** completely, honestly, and without interruptions.

**GENERAL HEALTH:**
**In general, would you say your health is:**
◯ Excellent    ◯Very Good    ◯Good    ◯Fair    ◯Poor

**Compared to one year ago, how would you rate your health in general now?**
◯ Much better now than one year ago
◯Somewhat better now than one year ago
◯About the same
◯Somewhat worse now than one year ago
◯Much worse than one year ago

**LIMITATIONS OF ACTIVITIES:**
The following items are about activities you might do during a typical day. Does your health now limit you in these activities? If so, how much?

**Vigorous activities, such as running, lifting heavy objects, participating in strenuous sports.**
◯Yes, Limited a lot    ◯Yes, Limited a Little    ◯No, Not Limited at all

**Moderate activities, such as moving a table, pushing a vacuum cleaner, bowling, or playing golf**
◯Yes, Limited a Lot    ◯Yes, Limited a Little    ◯No, Not Limited at all

**Lifting or carrying groceries**
◯Yes, Limited a Lot    ◯Yes, Limited a Little    ◯No, Not Limited at all

**Climbing several flights of stairs**
◯Yes, Limited a Lot    ◯Yes, Limited a Little    ◯No, Not Limited at all

**Climbing one flight of stairs**
◯Yes, Limited a Lot    ◯Yes, Limited a Little    ◯No, Not Limited at all

**Bending, kneeling, or stooping**
◯Yes, Limited a Lot    ◯Yes, Limited a Little    ◯No, Not Limited at all

**Walking more than a mile**
◯Yes, Limited a Lot    ◯Yes, Limited a Little    ◯No, Not Limited at all

**Walking several blocks**
◯Yes, Limited a Lot    ◯Yes, Limited a Little    ◯No, Not Limited at all

**Walking one block**
◯Yes, Limited a Lot    ◯Yes, Limited a Little    ◯No, Not Limited at all

**Bathing or dressing yourself**

◯ Yes, Limited a Lot          ◯ Yes, Limited a Little          ◯ No, Not Limited at all

**PHYSICAL HEALTH PROBLEMS:**
During the past 4 weeks, have you had any of the following problems with your work or other regular daily activities as a result of your physical health?

**Cut down the amount of time you spent on work or other activities**
◯ Yes          ◯ No

**Accomplished less than you would like**
◯ Yes          ◯ No

**Were limited in the kind of work or other activities**
◯ Yes          ◯ No

**Had difficulty performing the work or other activities (for example, it took extra effort)**
◯ Yes          ◯ No


**EMOTIONAL HEALTH PROBLEMS:**
During the past 4 weeks, have you had any of the following problems with your work or other regular daily activities as a result of any emotional problems (such as feeling depressed or anxious)?

**Cut down the amount of time you spent on work or other activities**
◯ Yes          ◯ No

**Accomplished less than you would like**
◯ Yes          ◯ No

**Didn't do work or other activities as carefully as usual**
◯ Yes          ◯ No

**SOCIAL ACTIVITIES:**
**Emotional problems interfered with your normal social activities with family, friends, neighbors, or groups?**

◯ Not at all          ◯ Slightly          ◯ Moderately          ◯ Severe          ◯ Very Severe

**PAIN:**
**How much bodily pain have you had during the past 4 weeks?**

◯ None          ◯ Very Mild          ◯ Mild          ◯ Moderate          ◯ Severe          ◯ Very Severe

**During the past 4 weeks, how much did pain interfere with your normal work (including both work outside the home and housework)?**

◯ Not at all          ◯ A little bit          ◯ Moderately          ◯ Quite a bit          ◯ Extremely

**ENERGY AND EMOTIONS:**
These questions are about how you feel and how things have been with you during the last 4 weeks. For each question, please give the answer that comes closest to the way you have been feeling.

**Did you feel full of pep?**
- All of the time
- Most of the time
- A good Bit of the Time
- Some of the time
- A little bit of the time
- None of the Time

**Have you been a very nervous person?**
- All of the time
- Most of the time
- A good Bit of the Time
- Some of the time
- A little bit of the time
- None of the Time

**Have you felt so down in the dumps that nothing could cheer you up?**
- All of the time
- Most of the time
- A good Bit of the Time
- Some of the time
- A little bit of the time
- None of the Time

**Have you felt calm and peaceful?**
- All of the time
- Most of the time
- A good Bit of the Time
- Some of the time
- A little bit of the time
- None of the Time

**Did you have a lot of energy?**
- All of the time
- Most of the time
- A good Bit of the Time
- Some of the time
- A little bit of the time
- None of the Time

**Have you felt downhearted and blue?**
◯ All of the time
◯ Most of the time
◯ A good Bit of the Time
◯ Some of the time
◯ A little bit of the time
◯ None of the Time

**Did you feel worn out?**
◯ All of the time
◯ Most of the time
◯ A good Bit of the Time
◯ Some of the time
◯ A little bit of the time
◯ None of the Time

**Have you been a happy person?**
◯ All of the time
◯ Most of the time
◯ A good Bit of the Time
◯ Some of the time
◯ A little bit of the time
◯ None of the Time

**Did you feel tired?**
◯ All of the time
◯ Most of the time
◯ A good Bit of the Time
◯ Some of the time
◯ A little bit of the time
◯ None of the Time

**SOCIAL ACTIVITIES:**
**During the past 4 weeks, how much of the time has your physical health or emotional problems interfered with your social activities (like visiting with friends, relatives, etc.)?**

◯ All of the time
◯ Most of the time
◯ Some of the time
◯ A little bit of the time
◯ None of the Time

**GENERAL HEALTH:**
**How true or false is each of the following statements for you?**

**I seem to get sick a little easier than other people**
◯ Definitely true    ◯ Mostly true    ◯ Don't know    ◯ Mostly false    ◯ Definitely false

**I am as healthy as anybody I know**
◯ Definitely true    ◯ Mostly true    ◯ Don't know    ◯ Mostly false    ◯ Definitely false

**I expect my health to get worse**
◯ Definitely true    ◯ Mostly true    ◯ Don't know    ◯ Mostly false    ◯ Definitely false

**My health is excellent**
◯ Definitely true    ◯ Mostly true    ◯ Don't know    ◯ Mostly false    ◯ Definitely false

Ware JE, Sherbourne CD. The MOS 36-Item Short Form Health Survey (SF-36). I: conceptual framework and item selection. Med Care. 1992;30(6):473-483. PMID: 1593914

# Short Form 12 (SF-12)

**SF-12 Health Survey**

This survey asks for your views about your health. This information will help keep track of how you feel and how well you are able to do your usual activities. **Answer each question by choosing just one answer**. If you are unsure how to answer a question, please give the best answer you can.

---

**1. In general, would you say your health is:**

☐₁ Excellent  ☐₂ Very good  ☐₃ Good  ☐₄ Fair  ☐₅ Poor

The following questions are about activities you might do during a typical day. Does <u>your health now limit you</u> in these activities? If so, how much?

| | YES, limited a lot | YES, limited a little | NO, not limited at all |
|---|---|---|---|
| 2. **Moderate activities** such as moving a table, pushing a vacuum cleaner, bowling, or playing golf. | ☐₁ | ☐₂ | ☐₃ |
| 3. Climbing **several** flights of stairs. | ☐₁ | ☐₂ | ☐₃ |

During the <u>past 4 weeks</u>, have you had any of the following problems with your work or other regular daily activities <u>as a result of your physical health</u>?

| | YES | NO |
|---|---|---|
| 4. **Accomplished less** than you would like. | ☐₁ | ☐₂ |
| 5. Were limited in the **kind** of work or other activities. | ☐₁ | ☐₂ |

During the <u>past 4 weeks</u>, have you had any of the following problems with your work or other regular daily activities <u>as a result of any emotional problems</u> (such as feeling depressed or anxious)?

| | YES | NO |
|---|---|---|
| 6. **Accomplished less** than you would like. | ☐₁ | ☐₂ |
| 7. Did work or activities **less carefully than usual**. | ☐₁ | ☐₂ |

8. During the <u>past 4 weeks</u>, how much <u>did pain interfere</u> with your normal work (including work outside the home and housework)?

☐₁ Not at all  ☐₂ A little bit  ☐₃ Moderately  ☐₄ Quite a bit  ☐₅ Extremely

These questions are about how you have been feeling during the <u>past 4 weeks</u>.
For each question, please give the one answer that comes closest to the way you have been feeling.

How much of the time during the <u>past 4 weeks</u>...

| | All of the time | Most of the time | A good bit of the time | Some of the time | A little of the time | None of the time |
|---|---|---|---|---|---|---|
| 9. Have you felt calm & peaceful? | ☐₁ | ☐₂ | ☐₃ | ☐₄ | ☐₅ | ☐₆ |
| 10. Did you have a lot of energy? | ☐₁ | ☐₂ | ☐₃ | ☐₄ | ☐₅ | ☐₆ |
| 11. Have you felt down-hearted and blue? | ☐₁ | ☐₂ | ☐₃ | ☐₄ | ☐₅ | ☐₆ |

12. During the <u>past 4 weeks</u>, how much of the time has your <u>physical health or emotional problems</u> interfered with your social activities (like visiting friends, relatives, etc.)?

☐₁ All of the time  ☐₂ Most of the time  ☐₃ Some of the time  ☐₄ A little of the time  ☐₅ None of the time

---

| Patient name: | Date: | PCS: | MCS: |
|---|---|---|---|

Visit type (circle one)
Preop    6 week    3 month    6 month    12 month    24 month    Other:__________

Ware J, Kosinski M, Keller SD. A 12-item short-form health survey: Construction of scales and preliminary tests of reliability and validity. Med Care 1996;34:220-233. DOI: https://doi.org/10.1097/00005650-199603000-00003

# Headache Disability Questionnaire (HDQ)

**HEADACHE DISABILITY QUESTIONNAIRE**

Name:.....................................        Date:........./........./..........        Score        / 90

**Please read each question and circle the response that best applies to you**

**1. How would you rate the usual pain of your headache on a scale from 0 to 10?**

| 0 | 1 | 2 | 3 | 4 | 5 | 6 | 7 | 8 | 9 | 10 | WORST |
|---|---|---|---|---|---|---|---|---|---|----|-------|

NO PAIN (under 0) — WORST PAIN (under 10)

**2. When you have headaches, how often is the pain severe?**

| NEVER | 1-9% | 10-19% | 20-29% | 30-39% | 40-49% | 50-59% | 60-69% | 70-79% | 80-89% | 90-100% | ALWAYS |
|-------|------|--------|--------|--------|--------|--------|--------|--------|--------|---------|--------|
| 0 | 1 | 2 | 3 | 4 | 5 | 6 | 7 | 8 | 9 | 10 | |

**3. On how many days in the last month did you actually lie down for an hour or more because of your headaches?**

| NONE | 1-3 | 4-6 | 7-9 | 10-12 | 13-15 | 16-18 | 19-21 | 22-24 | 25-27 | 28-31 | EVERY DAY |
|------|-----|-----|-----|-------|-------|-------|-------|-------|-------|-------|-----------|
| 0 | 1 | 2 | 3 | 4 | 5 | 6 | 7 | 8 | 9 | 10 | |

**4. When you have a headache, how often do you miss work or school for all or part of the day?**

| NEVER | 1-9% | 10-19% | 20-29% | 30-39% | 40-49% | 50-59% | 60-69% | 70-79% | 80-89% | 90-100% | ALWAYS |
|-------|------|--------|--------|--------|--------|--------|--------|--------|--------|---------|--------|
| 0 | 1 | 2 | 3 | 4 | 5 | 6 | 7 | 8 | 9 | 10 | |

**5. When you have a headache while you work (or school), how much is your ability to work reduced?**

| NOT | 1-9% | 10-19% | 20-29% | 30-39% | 40-49% | 50-59% | 60-69% | 70-79% | 80-89% | 90-100% | UNABLE |
|-----|------|--------|--------|--------|--------|--------|--------|--------|--------|---------|--------|
| 0 | 1 | 2 | 3 | 4 | 5 | 6 | 7 | 8 | 9 | 10 | TO WORK |

REDUCED (under 0)

**6. How many days in the last month have you been kept from performing housework or chores for at least half of the day because of your headaches?**

| NONE | 1-3 | 4-6 | 7-9 | 10-12 | 13-15 | 16-18 | 19-21 | 22-24 | 25-27 | 28-31 | EVERY DAY |
|------|-----|-----|-----|-------|-------|-------|-------|-------|-------|-------|-----------|
| 0 | 1 | 2 | 3 | 4 | 5 | 6 | 7 | 8 | 9 | 10 | |

**7. When you have a headache, how much is your ability to perform housework or chores reduced?**

| NOT | 1-9% | 10-19% | 20-29% | 30-39% | 40-49% | 50-59% | 60-69% | 70-79% | 80-89% | 90-100% | UNABLE |
|-----|------|--------|--------|--------|--------|--------|--------|--------|--------|---------|--------|
| 0 | 1 | 2 | 3 | 4 | 5 | 6 | 7 | 8 | 9 | 10 | TO PERFORM |

REDUCED (under 0)

**8. How many days in the last month have you been kept from non-work activities (family, social or recreational) because of your headaches?**

| NONE | 1-3 | 4-6 | 7-9 | 10-12 | 13-15 | 16-18 | 19-21 | 22-24 | 25-27 | 28-31 | EVERY DAY |
|------|-----|-----|-----|-------|-------|-------|-------|-------|-------|-------|-----------|
| 0 | 1 | 2 | 3 | 4 | 5 | 6 | 7 | 8 | 9 | 10 | |

**9. When you have a headache, how much is your ability to engage in non-work activities (family, social or recreational) reduced?**

| NOT | 1-9% | 10-19% | 20-29% | 30-39% | 40-49% | 50-59% | 60-69% | 70-79% | 80-89% | 90-100% | UNABLE |
|-----|------|--------|--------|--------|--------|--------|--------|--------|--------|---------|--------|
| 0 | 1 | 2 | 3 | 4 | 5 | 6 | 7 | 8 | 9 | 10 | TO PERFORM |

REDUCED (under 0)

K Niere, M Quin. Development of a headache-specific disability questionnaire for patients attending physiotherapy. Man Ther, 2009; 14:45-51. DOI: https://doi.org/10.1016/j.math.2007.09.006

# Migraine Interictal Burden Scale-4 (MIBS-4)

Please answer each of the following statements about the effect of your headaches in the past 4 weeks on days when you are not having an attack. **(X one box for each statement)**

Between headache attacks or at times when I do not have a headache

| | Don't know/NA | Never | Rarely | Some of the time | Much of the time | Most or all of the time |
|---|---|---|---|---|---|---|
| 1. My headaches affect my work or school at times when I do not have a headache | ☐ | ☐ | ☐ | ☐ | ☐ | ☐ |
| 2. I worry about planning social or leisure activities because I might have a headache | ☐ | ☐ | ☐ | ☐ | ☐ | ☐ |
| 3. My headaches impact my life at times when I do not have a headache | ☐ | ☐ | ☐ | ☐ | ☐ | ☐ |
| 4. At times when I do not have a headache, I feel helpless because of my headaches | ☐ | ☐ | ☐ | ☐ | ☐ | ☐ |
| Total number of checks in column | | | | | | |
| Multiply number of checks by value = total score per column | x0 | x0 | x1 | x2 | x3 | x3 |
| Total score per column | | | | | | |
| Total score | + | + | + | + | + | = |

**MIBS-4 scoring key**

| Score | Level of interictal burden | Treatment recommendations |
|---|---|---|
| 0 | None | • No action needed |
| 1-2 | Mild | • Offer non-pharmacological strategies for reducing interictal burden<br>• Offer/optimize acute pharmacological treatment |
| 3-4 | Moderate | • Offer non-pharmacological strategies for reducing interictal burden<br>• Offer/optimize acute pharmacological treatment<br>• Consider preventive pharmacological treatment |
| 5+ | Severe | • Offer non-pharmacological strategies for reducing interictal burden<br>• Offer/optimize acute pharmacological treatment<br>• Offer preventive pharmacological treatment |

Buse DC, Bigal MB, Rupnow M, Reed M, Serrano D, Lipton RB: Development and validation of the Migraine Interictal Burden Scale (MIBS): a self-administered instrument for measuring the burden of migraine between attacks (abstract S05.003). Neurology. 2007;68(suppl 1):A89.

# Migraine Specific Quality of Life Questionnaire (Version 2.1)

> While answering the following questions, please think about *all migraine attacks* you may have had *in the past 4 weeks*.

1.In the <u>past 4 weeks</u>, how often have migraines **interfered** with how well you dealt with family, friends and others who are close to you? (Select only **one** response.)

- ₁❏ None of the time
- ₂❏ A little bit of the time
- ₃❏ Some of the time
- ₄❏ A good bit of the time
- ₅❏ Most of the time
- ₆❏ All of the time

2. In the <u>past 4 weeks</u>, how often have migraines **interfered** with your leisure time activities, such as reading or exercising? (Select only **one** response.)

- ₁❏ None of the time
- ₂❏ A little bit of the time
- ₃❏ Some of the time
- ₄❏ A good bit of the time
- ₅❏ Most of the time
- ₆❏ All of the time

3. In the <u>past 4 weeks</u>, how often have you had **difficulty** in performing work or daily activities because of migraine symptoms? (Select only **one** response.)

- ₁❏ None of the time
- ₂❏ A little bit of the time
- ₃❏ Some of the time
- ₄❏ A good bit of the time
- ₅❏ Most of the time
- ₆❏ All of the time

4. In the <u>past 4 weeks</u>, how often did migraines **keep you** from getting as much done at work or at home? (Select only **one** response.)

- ₁❏ None of the time
- ₂❏ A little bit of the time
- ₃❏ Some of the time
- ₄❏ A good bit of the time
- ₅❏ Most of the time
- ₆❏ All of the time

5. In the <u>past 4 weeks</u>, how often did migraines **limit** your ability to concentrate on work or daily activities? (Select only **one** response.)

$_1$❑ None of the time
$_2$❑ A little bit of the time
$_3$❑ Some of the time
$_4$❑ A good bit of the time
$_5$❑ Most of the time
$_6$❑ All of the time

6. In the <u>past 4 weeks</u>, how often have migraines **left you too tired** to do work or daily activities? (Select only **one** response.)

$_1$❑ None of the time
$_2$❑ A little bit of the time
$_3$❑ Some of the time
$_4$❑ A good bit of the time
$_5$❑ Most of the time
$_6$❑ All of the time

7. In the <u>past 4 weeks</u>, how often have migraines **limited** the number of days you have felt energetic? (Select only **one** response.)

$_1$❑ None of the time
$_2$❑ A little bit of the time
$_3$❑ Some of the time
$_4$❑ A good bit of the time
$_5$❑ Most of the time
$_6$❑ All of the time

8. In the <u>past 4 weeks</u>, how often have you had to **cancel** work or daily activities because you had a migraine? (Select only **one** response.)

$_1$❑ None of the time
$_2$❑ A little bit of the time
$_3$❑ Some of the time
$_4$❑ A good bit of the time
$_5$❑ Most of the time
$_6$❑ All of the time

9. In the <u>past 4 weeks</u>, how often did you **need help** in handling routine tasks such as every day household chores, doing necessary business, shopping, or caring for others, when you had a migraine? (Select only **one** response.)

$_1$❑ None of the time
$_2$❑ A little bit of the time
$_3$❑ Some of the time
$_4$❑ A good bit of the time
$_5$❑ Most of the time
$_6$❑ All of the time

10. In the <u>past 4 weeks</u>, how often did you have to **stop** work or daily activities to deal with migraine symptoms? (Select only **one** response.)

₁❑ None of the time
₂❑ A little bit of the time
₃❑ Some of the time
₄❑ A good bit of the time
₅❑ Most of the time
₆❑ All of the time

11. In the <u>past 4 weeks</u>, how often were you **not able to go** to social activities such as parties, dinner with friends, because you had a migraine? (Select only **one** response.)

₁❑ None of the time
₂❑ A little bit of the time
₃❑ Some of the time
₄❑ A good bit of the time
₅❑ Most of the time
₆❑ All of the time

12. In the <u>past 4 weeks</u>, how often have you **felt** fed up or frustrated because of your migraines? (Select only **one** response.)

₁❑ None of the time
₂❑ A little bit of the time
₃❑ Some of the time
₄❑ A good bit of the time
₅❑ Most of the time
₆❑ All of the time

13. In the <u>past 4 weeks</u>, how often have you **felt** like you were a burden on others because of your migraines? (Select only **one** response.)

₁❑ None of the time
₂❑ A little bit of the time
₃❑ Some of the time
₄❑ A good bit of the time
₅❑ Most of the time
₆❑ All of the time

14. In the <u>past 4 weeks</u>, how often have you been **afraid** of letting others down because of your migraines? (Select only **one** response.)

₁❑ None of the time
₂❑ A little bit of the time
₃❑ Some of the time
₄❑ A good bit of the time
₅❑ Most of the time
₆❑ All of the time

Jhidran P, Osterhaus JT, Miller DW, Lee JT, Kirchdoerfer L. Development and validation of the Migraine-Specific Quality of Life Questionnaire. Headache 1998;38:295-302. DOI: https://doi.org/10.1046/j.1526-4610.1998.3804295.x

# Red and Orange Flags for Secondary Headaches in Clinical Practice

**Table 1** SNNOOP10 list of red and orange flags

| | Sign or symptom | Related secondary headaches (most relevant ICHD-3b categories) | Flag color |
|---|---|---|---|
| 1 | Systemic symptoms including fever | Headache attributed to infection or nonvascular intracranial disorders, carcinoid or pheochromocytoma | Red (orange for isolated fever) |
| 2 | Neoplasm in history | Neoplasms of the brain; metastasis | Red |
| 3 | Neurologic deficit or dysfunction (including decreased consciousness) | Headaches attributed to vascular, nonvascular intracranial disorders; brain abscess and other infections | Red |
| 4 | Onset of headache is sudden or abrupt | Subarachnoid hemorrhage and other headaches attributed to cranial or cervical vascular disorders | Red |
| 5 | Older age (after 50 years) | Giant cell arteritis and other headache attributed to cranial or cervical vascular disorders; neoplasms and other nonvascular intracranial disorders | Red |
| 6 | Pattern change or recent onset of headache | Neoplasms, headaches attributed to vascular, nonvascular intracranial disorders | Red |
| 7 | Positional headache | Intracranial hypertension or hypotension | Red |
| 8 | Precipitated by sneezing, coughing, or exercise | Posterior fossa malformations; Chiari malformation | Red |
| 9 | Papilledema | Neoplasms and other nonvascular intracranial disorders; intracranial hypertension | Red |
| 10 | Progressive headache and atypical presentations | Neoplasms and other nonvascular intracranial disorders | Red |
| 11 | Pregnancy or puerperium | Headaches attributed to cranial or cervical vascular disorders; postdural puncture headache; hypertension-related disorders (e.g., preeclampsia); cerebral sinus thrombosis; hypothyroidism; anemia; diabetes | Red |
| 12 | Painful eye with autonomic features | Pathology in posterior fossa, pituitary region, or cavernous sinus; Tolosa-Hunt syndrome; ophthalmic causes | Red |
| 13 | Posttraumatic onset of headache | Acute and chronic posttraumatic headache; subdural hematoma and other headache attributed to vascular disorders | Red |
| 14 | Pathology of the immune system such as HIV | Opportunistic infections | Red |
| 15 | Painkiller overuse or new drug at onset of headache | Medication overuse headache; drug incompatibility | Red |

Thien Phu Do, MD, Angelique Remmers, MD, Henrik Winther Schytz, MD, PhD, DMSc, Christoph Schankin, MD, Sarah E. Nelson, MD, Mark Obermann, MD, Jakob Møller Hansen, MD, PhD, Alexandra J. Sinclair, MD, PhD, Andreas R. Gantenbein, MD, and Guus G. Schoonman, MD, PhD. Red and orange flags for secondary headaches in clinical practice SNNOOP10 list. Neurology ® 2019;92:134–144. https://doi.org/10.1212/WNL.0000000000006697.

# The SNNOOP10 List of Red Flags

|   | Sign or symptom | Related secondary etiology | Key points |
|---|---|---|---|
| 1 | Systemic symptoms including fever | Headache attributed to infection or non-vascular intracranial disorders, carcinoid or pheochromocytoma. | Headache with fever is primarily alarming when accompanied by relevant symptoms (e.g., neck stiffness, decreased consciousness, and neurologic deficit). |
| 2 | Neoplasm in history | Neoplasms of the brain; metastasis. | A newly developed headache in a patient with neoplasm is highly suspect for an intracranial metastasis. |
| 3 | Neurological deficit or dysfunction (including decreased consciousness) | Headaches attributed to vascular, non-vascular intracranial disorders. Brain abscess and other infections. | Headache occurs in one-fourth of episodes of acute stroke. The severity of headache is not related to the size of the lesion. |
| 4 | Onset of headache is sudden or abrupt (thunderclap headache) | Subarachnoid hemorrhage and other headaches attributed to cranial or cervical vascular disorders. | Thunderclap headache can be the only initial symptom of subarachnoid hemorrhage. |
| 5 | Older age (after 50 years) | Giant cell arteritis and other headache attributed to cranial or cervical vascular disorders. Neoplasms and other non-vascular intracranial disorders. | Older individuals with headache have a higher frequency of secondary etiology. The incidence of primary headache disorders is also lower in this age group. |
| 6 | Pattern change or recent onset of headache | Neoplasms, headaches attributed to vascular, non-vascular intracranial disorders. | A recent change of pattern or a newly developed headache can be the only signs of a secondary etiology. Diagnosis is often delayed in these cases. |
| 7 | Positional headache | Intracranial hypertension or hypotension. | Positional headache is the trademark of intracranial hypotension, and the most common cause is cerebrospinal fluid leak at the spinal level. |
| 8 | Precipitated by sneezing, coughing or exercise | Posterior fossa lesions, Chiari malformation. | Cough headache is highly predictive of Chiari malformations and posterior fossa lesions. |
| 9 | Papilledema | Neoplasms and other non-vascular intracranial disorders; intracranial hypertension. | A high prevalence of patients with papilledema has a serious underlying pathology. |
| 10 | Progressive headache and atypical presentations | Neoplasms and other non-vascular intracranial disorders. | Progressive headache and atypical headache presentation can be the only signs of serious underlying pathology. |

|    | Sign or symptom | Related secondary etiology | Key points |
|----|-----------------|----------------------------|------------|
| 11 | Pregnancy or puerperium | Headaches attributed to cranial or cervical vascular disorders; post-dural puncture headache; hypertension related disorders (e.g., preeclampsia); cerebral venous thrombosis; hypothyroidism; anemia; diabetes. | Headache during pregnancy and puerperium has a higher risk of severe pathology. More than one-third of individuals presenting to acute care with headache during pregnancy will have a secondary etiology. Most common causes are hypertensive disorders followed by pituitary adenoma or stroke. Other risk factors are no prior headache history, occurring during third trimester, seizures, hypertension, and fever. |
| 12 | Painful eye with autonomic features | Pathology in posterior fossa, pituitary region or cavernous sinus. Tolosa-Hunt syndrome. Ophthalmic causes. | Patients with presentations of painful eye with autonomic features should undergo neuroimaging as it can be due to a structural lesion. Even typical presentations of cluster headache (or other trigeminal autonomic cephalalgias) can derive from a structural lesion. |
| 13 | Posttraumatic onset of headache | Acute and chronic posttraumatic headache; subdural hematoma and other headache attributed to vascular disorders. | Headache related to trauma should always be explored. |
| 14 | Pathology of the immune system such as AIDS (acquired immunodeficiency syndrome)) or medical immunosuppression | Opportunistic infections. | Risk of severe pathology is dependent on the degree of immunosuppression. |
| 15 | Painkiller overuse or new drug at onset of headache | Medication overuse headache; drug incompatibility. | Medication overuse is the most common cause of secondary headache. Onset of headache due to a new drug can be a sign of incompatibility with the given drug. |

Red flags are information that encourage further investigation of a secondary etiology.

# Green Flags for Headache Disorders

|   | Sign or symptom | Key points |
|---|---|---|
| 1 | The current headache has already been present during childhood | Viral infections are the most common cause of secondary headache in children. In children with chronic headache, the pain is rarely secondary. A life-threatening headache is very unlikely in adults in whom that headache type has already been present during childhood. |
| 2 | The patient has headache-free days | Most primary headache disorders are paroxysmal. Although recurring secondary headache also occur, they are often caused by trigger factors, such as injury to the head, cerebral ischemia, intracranial hemorrhage, arteritis, arterial dissection, or exposure to a substance, e.g., phosphodiesterase inhibitors or nitric oxide donors. An important exception are intracranial tumors that can also present with recurring headache. |
| 3 | The headache occurs in temporal relationship with the menstrual cycle | The relationship between pain and menstrual cycle has been validated with a headache diary. Migraine attacks associated with fluctuations in the menstrual cycle is common. |
| 4 | Close family members have the same headache phenotype | There is a genetic disposition to migraine, cluster headache, and medication overuse headache. The prevalence of genetic vasculopathies is lower than the beforementioned headache disorders. |
| 5 | Headache occurred or stopped more than 1 week ago | Life-threatening secondary headache generally present within few days. Consequently, the more time passed since the headache, the smaller the probability of a life-threatening cause. However, time passed since onset is unlikely to influence the likelihood of other non-life-threatening secondary causes, e.g., temporomandibular disorder, persistent post-traumatic headache. |

Green flags are information that may suggest that no further investigations for a secondary etiology is needed.

## ID Migraine Screener

| During the past 3 months, did you have the following with your headaches? | |
| --- | --- |
| 1 | You felt nauseated or sick to your stomach? |
| Yes | No |
| 2 | Light bothered you (a lot more than when you don't have headaches)? |
| Yes | No |
| 3 | Your headaches limited your ability to work, study, or do what you needed to do? |
| Yes | No |

The three-item ID Migraine Screener interrogates on nausea, photophobia, and disability. It is positive if ≥2 items are fulfilled.

Lipton RB, Dodick D, Sadovsky R, Kolodner K, Endicott J, Hettiarachchi J, et al. A self- administered screener for migraine in primary care. The IDMigraine™ validation study. Neurology. 2003;61:375–382.

## Migraine Screen Questionnaire

| INSTRUCTIONS: The questions below refer to the headaches or migraine episodes without headache that you may have experienced in your lifetime. Answer each question as indicated. If you are not sure how to answer a given question, please answer what you believe is most correct. | |
| --- | --- |
| 1 | Do you have frequent or intense headaches? |
| Yes | No |
| 2 | Do your headaches usually last more than 4 h? |
| Yes | No |
| 3 | Do you usually suffer from nausea when you have a headache? |
| Yes | No |
| 4 | Does light or noise bother you when you have a headache? |
| Yes | No |
| 5 | Does headache limit any of your physical or intellectual activities? |
| Yes | No |

Láinez MJ, Castillo J, Domínguez M, Palacios G, Díaz S, Rejas J. New uses of the Migraine Screen Questionnaire (MS-Q): validation in the Primary Care setting and ability to detect hidden migraine. MS-Q in Primary Care. BMC Neurology 2010;10:39.

## The Erwin Test for Cluster Headache

| The Erwin test for cluster headache | |
| --- | --- |
| 1 | Is this the worst pain you have ever experienced? |
| Yes | No |
| 2 | Imagine setting a timer. Does the last less than 4 h? |
| Yes | No |
| 3 | During a headache, do one or more of these happen to you?<br>• your eye turns red on only one side<br>• your eye waters on only one side<br>• your nose runs on only one side<br>• your nose gets congested on only one side |
| Yes | No |

Parakramaweera R, Evans RE, Schor LI, Pearson SM, Martines R, Cammarata, et al. A brief diagnostic screen for cluster headache: Creation and initial validation of the Erwin Test for Cluster Headache Cephalalgia 2021;41(13):1298–1309.

## Wong-Baker Faces Pain Rating Scales

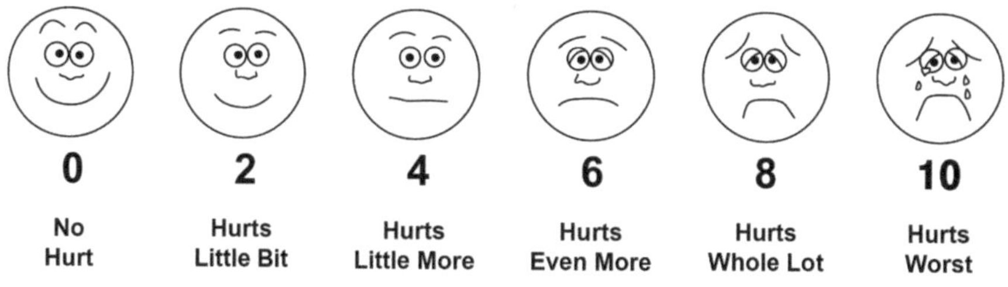

# Headache-Attributed Lost Time (HALT-90) Index

## Lifting The Burden
### The Global Campaign against Headache

A collaboration between the World Health Organization,
non-governmental organisations, academic institutions and individuals worldwide

### HALT Index*
(Headache-Attributed Lost Time)

**Your doctor or nurse may give you this short questionnaire before starting treatment.**

**Please answer the five simple questions. This will help your doctor or nurse understand how much your headaches are affecting your life, and guide your medical treatment.**

### Please answer these five questions carefully

1. On how many **days** in the **last three months** could you **not go** to work or school because of your headaches?

2. On how many **days** in the **last three months** could you do **less than half** your usual amount in your job or schoolwork because of your headaches? (Do not include days you counted in question 1 where you missed work or school.)

3. On how many **days** in the **last three months** could you **not do any** household work because of your headaches?

4. On how many **days** in the **last three months** could you do **less than half** your usual amount of household work because of your headaches? (Do not include days you counted in question 3 where you did not do household work.)

5. On how many **days** in the **last three months** did you **miss** family, social or leisure activities because of your headaches?

**Grading** (I-IV indicate, in order, increasing need for medical care; either III or IV indicates high need)

| | | |
|---|---|---|
| 0-5 | Minimal or infrequent impact | Grade I |
| 6-10 | Mild or infrequent impact | Grade II |
| 11-20 | Moderate impact | Grade III |
| 20+ | Severe impact | Grade IV |

**TOTAL**

* HALT is closely based on the first five questions of MIDAS, developed by RB Lipton and WF Stewart

Steiner TJ., Lipton RB, and on behalf of Lifting the Burden: The Global Campaign against Headache. The Journal of Headache and Pain, 2018;19:12. doi: https://doi.org/10.1186/s10194-018-0837-3

# HARDSHIP Questionnaire

**Additional file 1. The HARDSHIP questionnaire**

## *Lifting The Burden*

**in Official Relations with
the World Health Organization**

**The Global Campaign against Headache**

### Headache-attributed restriction, disability, social handicap and impaired participation (HARDSHIP) questionnaire

**for administration by medical or trained lay interviewers
to population samples**

<table>
<tr><td>Centre identifier<br>(to be completed by the centre)</td><td>_____________________________</td></tr>
<tr><td colspan="2">Participant identifier<br>(to be completed by the interviewer)</td></tr>
<tr><td colspan="2">

☐  ☐ ☐ ☐  ☐ ☐ ☐  ☐ ☐

enter letter to identify stratum:

  U: urban<br>  S: semi-rural<br>  R: rural

from master lists of sampling units and households:

  enter 3-digit number to identify sampling unit followed by 3-digit number to identify household within sampling unit

from occupant list on next page:

enter 2-digit number to identify household occupant

</td></tr>
<tr><td>Interviewer identifier<br>(to be completed by the interviewer)<br><br>_____________________</td><td>Interviewer signature (on completion):</td></tr>
</table>

## Participant identification

| Address of household and name of head of household<br><br>[not required if the survey data are to remain anonymous] | | | | |
|---|---|---|---|---|

|  |  | Given name | Age (y) | M/F |
|---|---|---|---|---|
| | **01** | | | |
| | **02** | | | |
| | **03** | | | |
| | **04** | | | |
| | **05** | | | |
| Numbered list of household occupants<br><br>(enter given name, age and gender of each occupant in the order supplied)<br><br>(age may be estimated if the date of birth is unknown) | **06** | | | |
| | **07** | | | |
| | **08** | | | |
| | **09** | | | |
| | **10** | | | |
| | **11** | | | |
| | **12** | | | |
| | **13** | | | |
| | **14** | | | |

Select one occupant at random from the total number of occupants: the selected person will be the participant.

Enter the number in the next column and on the previous page.

☐☐

enter number to identify selected household occupant

Thank you for answering the following questions. Please begin by entering **today's date**, and then answer **all questions on this day**.

| 1 | Please enter today's date | _______ / _______ / _________ |

## Demographic questions

| 2 | What is your age? | _______ years |
| 3 | What is your gender?<br>(please tick one box) | male ☐   female ☐ |

## Social situation questions

| 4 | What is your marital status?<br>(please tick one box **only**) | ☐ single   ☐ married   ☐ widow or widower   ☐ separated or divorced |
| 5 | Are you living with a household partner?<br>(please tick one box)<br><br>(a household partner may be husband or wife, or an unmarried partner of either gender in a stable relationship) | no ☐   yes ☐ |
| 6 | Which of these is closest to your personal situation?<br>(please tick one box **only**) | ☐ **employed or self-employed** (go to question 7)<br><br>☐ **homemaker or housewife** (go to question 8)   ☐ **student** (go to question 8)   ☐ **unemployed** (go to question 8)   ☐ **retired** (go to question 8) |

<table>
<tr>
<td>7</td>
<td>Which of these best describes your work?<br>(please tick one box only)<br><br>[the categories listed are suggestions; they should be adapted and/or supplemented as appropriate for the country]</td>
<td>professional ☐<br><br>semi-professional ☐<br><br>skilled worker ☐<br><br>semi-skilled worker ☐<br><br>unskilled worker ☐</td>
</tr>
<tr>
<td>8</td>
<td>What is your total net household income per year?<br>(please tick one box)<br><br>[the values of W, X, Y and Z in national currency units (NCU) should correspond to the national household income quintiles, so that one fifth of the population falls into each income category; as an alternative, the question may relate to personal income and W, X, Y and Z should then correspond to national per capita income quintiles]</td>
<td>less than NCU W ☐<br><br>between NCU W+1 and NCU X ☐<br><br>between NCU X+1 and NCU Y ☐<br><br>between NCU Y+1 and NCU Z ☐<br><br>more than NCU Z ☐</td>
</tr>
<tr>
<td>9</td>
<td>How many years did you complete in full-time education?<br>(please add together all the years at school or places of higher education)</td>
<td>_______ years</td>
</tr>
<tr>
<td>10</td>
<td>What is your native language (the language you first learned to speak)?</td>
<td>enter name of language:</td>
</tr>
<tr>
<td>11</td>
<td>What language do you usually speak in your own home?<br><br>[this question may, if appropriate, be replaced or supplemented by questions on ethnicity]</td>
<td>enter name of language:</td>
</tr>
</table>

| **Screen questions** | | |
|---|---|---|
| **12** | Have you **ever** had a headache **in your lifetime?**<br>(please tick one box) | no ☐　　yes ☐ |
| **13** | Have you had a headache **during the last 12 months?**<br>(please tick one box) | no ☐　　yes ☐<br><br>(if no, go directly to question 87) |
| **14** | During **the last 30 days**, on how many of these days did you have a headache?<br>(please enter number of days between 0 and 30) | ________ days<br><br>(if you answered between 15 and 30 days, please continue with question 15; otherwise, go directly to question 19) |

### "Daily" headache questions

You have said that you had headache **on 15 or more days in the last month**. Please think about these headaches.

| | | |
|---|---|---|
| **15** | How long do these headaches usually last?<br>(please enter the number of minutes or hours, or tick the box) | ☐<br>never goes away<br>______ min or ______ hr |
| **16** | Do you take **any medication to treat** these headaches?<br>(please tick one box)<br><br>(please note that this question is about treatment to **relieve** the headache, not daily treatment to **prevent** headache) | no ☐　　yes ☐<br><br>(if no, go directly to question 19) |
| **17** | What medication **do you use most** to treat these headaches?<br><br>and what other medications do you also take for this purpose?<br>(if there are no others, please write "none")<br><br>(please note that this question is only about treatment to **relieve** headache) | name the most-used medication:<br><br>list all other medications: |
| **18** | Altogether, on how many days in the last 30 days did you take these medications?<br>(please enter number of days between 0 and 30) | ________ days |

## "Most bothersome headache" questions

These are questions on the headaches that interfere most with your life. These headaches may be the same as the headaches you have just described, or they may be different headaches if you have more than one type of headache.

| 19 | Please think about your headaches. Do you think they **are all of one type**, or are they of **more than one type**? (please tick one box) | one ☐        more than one ☐ |

If you answered one, the next questions are to diagnose this headache. Please start at question 20.

If you answered more than one, from now on please focus upon the headache type that on the whole bothers you most (*ie*, interferes most with your life).

The next series of questions are intended to diagnose <u>this</u> type of headache. Please start at question 20.

## Diagnostic questions

| 20 | How often do you have **this type of headache**? (please tick box or enter the number of days per month or per year) | ☐  ______  ______<br>**every day   days/month   days/year** |
| 21 | How long does **this type of headache usually last**? (please enter the number of minutes, hours or days, or tick the box) (if the headache goes away during sleep, count the time until you wake up without it) | ____ mins, ____ hours or ____ days<br><br>**never goes away** ☐ |
| 22 | Is your last answer **with or without** medication? (please tick one box) | **with** ☐        **without** ☐<br><br>(if you answered "without medication", please go to question 24) |
| 23 | How long would it last **if you did not take medication**? (please enter the number of minutes, hours or days) | ____ mins, ____ hours or ____ days |
| 24 | How bad is **this type of headache** usually? (please tick one box) | ☐         ☐         ☐<br>**not bad   quite bad   very bad** |

| 25 | There are many ways of describing a headache, but most are either throbbing or pressing.<br><br>Thinking still of **this type of headache**, which best describes the pain?<br>(please tick one box) | ☐ **throbbing or pulsating** (this means varying in time with the heart beat)     ☐ **pressing, squeezing or tightening** |
|---|---|---|
| 26 | Is the pain of **this type of headache** usually on only one side of the head?<br>(please tick one box) | **no** ☐    **yes** ☐ |
| 27 | Does exercise (like walking or climbing stairs) tend to make it worse?<br>(please tick one box) | **no** ☐    **yes** ☐ |
| 28 | Thinking still of **this type of headache**, how does it affect your ability to do day-to-day activities?<br>(please tick one box) | ☐ **can do everything as normal**    ☐ **cannot do some things**    ☐ **can do nothing** |
| 29 | With **this type of headache**, do you usually feel nauseated (as though you may vomit or throw up)?<br>(please tick one box) | **no** ☐    **yes** ☐ |
| 30 | With **this type of headache**, do you usually actually vomit (throw up)?<br>(please tick one box) | **no** ☐    **yes** ☐ |
| 31 | When you have **this type of headache**, does daylight or other lighting bother you? In other words, do you prefer to be in the dark?<br>(please tick one box) | ☐ **no**    ☐ **not sure**    ☐ **yes**<br><br>(this question refers to <u>ordinary</u> levels of light, not bright lighting) |
| 32 | When you have **this type of headache**, does noise bother you? In other words, do you prefer to be in the quiet?<br>(please tick one box) | ☐ **no**    ☐ **not sure**    ☐ **yes**<br><br>(this question refers to <u>ordinary</u> levels of noise, not very loud noise) |

<table>
<tr><td>33</td><td>Has a health-care professional ever given you a diagnosis for this type of headache?<br>(please tick one box and, if yes, enter the diagnosis)</td><td>no ☐    yes ☐<br><br>If yes, please write the diagnosis:</td></tr>
</table>

The next series of questions are specifically about **yesterday** (the day before you fill in your answers).

It is very important that the answers you give are about **yesterday** and not any other day.

### Questions about yesterday

<table>
<tr><td>34</td><td>Did you have a headache yesterday?<br>(please tick one box)</td><td>no ☐    yes ☐<br><br>(if no, go directly to question 46)</td></tr>
<tr><td>35</td><td>Was this the type of headache you have just been describing?<br>(please tick one box)</td><td>no ☐    yes ☐</td></tr>
<tr><td>36</td><td>Please think about the headache you had yesterday. How long did it last?<br>(please tick the box if it was present all day, from waking in the morning until bedtime, or enter the number of hours between 1 and 24)</td><td>all day ☐ or ______ hours</td></tr>
<tr><td>37</td><td>How bad was this headache yesterday?<br>(please tick one box)</td><td>☐    ☐    ☐<br>not bad   quite bad   very bad</td></tr>
<tr><td>38</td><td>Please think about everything you wanted to do yesterday if you had not had a headache.<br><br>How much of this did you actually do?<br>(please tick one box)</td><td>☐    ☐    ☐    ☐<br>nothing   less than half   more than half   everything</td></tr>
<tr><td>39</td><td>Was yesterday a workday (either at your job or at school)?<br>(please tick one box)</td><td>no ☐    yes ☐<br><br>(if no, go directly to question 43)</td></tr>
</table>

**40** Because of your headache, did you miss work or school **yesterday**? (please tick one box or enter the number of hours lost from work or school)

☐ no

arrived late, took time out during the day or left early (please enter the total number of hours lost):

__________ hours

☐ missed the whole day (please go to question 42)

**41** If you were at work or school with your **headache yesterday**, how much of your work did you get done? (please tick one box))

☐ nothing  ☐ less than half  ☐ more than half  ☐ everything (please go to question 43)

**42** Will you able to make up for this today or later? (please tick one box)

☐ no  ☐ partly  ☐ completely

**43** Please think about household work or general chores that you wanted to do **yesterday** if you had not had headache.

How much of this did you **actually do**? (please tick one box)

☐ nothing  ☐ less than half  ☐ more than half  ☐ everything

**44** Please think about leisure and social activities that you wanted to do **yesterday** if you had not had headache.

How much of this did you **actually do**? (please tick one box)

☐ nothing  ☐ less than half  ☐ more than half  ☐ everything

**45** What treatment did you take for the **headache you had yesterday**?

Please tick the box if you took nothing; otherwise, please list the names of all medications taken for headache yesterday, and the number of times each was taken yesterday.

nothing at all ☐

**List medications:** (please list medications for **headache**, not for any other illnesses)

how many times you took each

________________________________   ________

________________________________   ________

________________________________   ________

________________________________   ________

________________________________   ________

## Health care questions

The aim of the following questions is to help us know how much health care should be available to meet the needs of people with headache.

**46** Many different medications may be used successfully to treat headache.

Some are prescription-only, whilst others can be bought over the counter.

Please look at these lists. Which of these have you used **in the last month?**

Please tick the box if you took nothing at all in the whole of the last month; otherwise, enter by each medication the number of days on which you used it in the last month.

[This question is country-specific, and the list should be adapted as appropriate]

nothing at all ☐

number of days

almotriptan (Almogran) ______

eletriptan (Relpax) ______

frovatriptan (Migard) ______

naratriptan (Naramig) ______

rizatriptan (Maxalt) ______

sumatriptan (Imigran) ______

zolmitriptan (Zomig) ______

ergotamine (Cafergot, Migril) ______

domperidone (Motilium) ______

metoclopramide (Maxolon, Primperan) ______

aspirin (acetylsalicylic acid) ______

diclofenac (Voltarol) ______

ibuprofen (Nurofen) ______

ketoprofen (Ketocid, Orudis) ______

mefenamic acid (Ponstan) ______

naproxen (Naprosyn) ______

paracetamol (Panadol) ______

tolfenamic acid (Clotam) ______

Proprietary combination drugs:

Excedrin ______

Migraleve ______

Migramax ______

Nuromol ______

Paramax ______

Solpadeine ______

Syndol ______

<table>
<tr>
<td>46<br>(cont)</td>
<td>Are there any other medications you have used to treat your headache in the last month?<br><br>Please enter the name of each other medication and, by each, the number of days on which you used it in the last month.</td>
<td>Name(s) of medication(s):<br>(please list medications for headache, not for any other illnesses)<br><br>____________________<br>____________________<br>____________________<br>____________________<br>____________________<br>____________________</td>
<td>number of days<br><br>____<br>____<br>____<br>____<br>____<br>____</td>
</tr>
<tr>
<td>47</td>
<td>Medications to prevent headaches are usually taken daily. Are you taking any of these now?<br><br>Please enter the name(s) and, by each one, for how long in weeks or months you have been taking it.</td>
<td>Name(s) of medication(s):<br><br>____________________<br>____________________<br>____________________</td>
<td>how long taken?<br><br>____<br>____<br>____</td>
</tr>
<tr>
<td>48</td>
<td>Many people with headache treat themselves, but others need professional advice.<br><br>Have you had professional advice about your headaches in the last year? Who from, and how many times?<br><br>Please tick all boxes that apply and, for each ticked box, enter the number of times in the last year.<br><br>[Other categories may be added or substituted when relevant to the country]</td>
<td>no-one ☐<br><br>nurse ☐<br><br>physical therapist (physiotherapist, osteopath, chiropractor) ☐<br><br>clinical officer ☐<br><br>primary-care doctor (GP) ☐<br><br>headache specialist ☐<br><br>ear, nose and throat doctor ☐<br><br>eye doctor ☐<br><br>hospital emergency room ☐<br><br>other (please specify): ☐<br>____________________</td>
<td>number of times<br><br>____<br>____<br>____<br>____<br>____<br>____<br>____<br>____<br>____</td>
</tr>
</table>

| | | |
|---|---|---|
| **49** | Most people with headache do not require any investigations, but occasionally these tests are done.<br><br>Because of your headaches, have you had any of these tests **in the last year**?<br>(please tick <u>all</u> that apply)<br><br>[Other country-relevant investigations, such as blood smear for malaria, may be added] | **MRI brain scan** ☐<br><br>**CT brain scan** ☐<br><br>**x-rays of the neck** ☐<br><br>**eye tests (for glasses)** ☐<br><br>**blood tests** ☐ |
| **50** | Have you, **in the last year**, been admitted to hospital **because of your headaches**?<br>(please tick one box and, if yes, enter the total number of days in hospital) | **no** ☐　　**yes** ☐<br><br>**total number of days** ______ |

## Impact questions

The next questions are about the effects your headaches have on **your own life**.

| | | |
|---|---|---|
| **51** | Have your headaches interfered with your **education**?<br>(please tick all boxes that apply **because of your headaches**) | ☐ **no**　☐ **yes, I did less well**　☐ **yes, I did not attempt something**　☐ **yes, I gave up early** |
| **52** | Do you believe your headaches have made you less successful in your career?<br>(please tick all boxes that apply **because of your headaches**)<br><br>(if this question is not applicable to you, please tick no and go directly to question 54) | **no** ☐<br><br>**yes, I have done less well** ☐<br><br>**yes, I have attempted less** ☐<br><br>**yes, I have taken an easier job** ☐<br><br>**yes, I have taken long-term sick leave** ☐<br><br>**yes, I have retired early** ☐<br><br>**yes, I am on a disability pension** ☐ |

| 53 | Have your headaches reduced your **earnings**? (please tick one box) | no ☐    yes ☐ |
|---|---|---|

| 54 | Do you feel that your employer and work colleagues understand and accept your headaches? (please tick one box) | ☐ no    ☐ partly    ☐ yes, fully |
|---|---|---|

| 55 | Do you feel that your family and friends understand and accept your headaches? (please tick one box) | ☐ no    ☐ partly    ☐ yes, fully |
|---|---|---|

| 56 | Do you avoid telling people that you have headaches? (please tick one box) | no ☐    yes ☐ |
|---|---|---|

| 57 | Taking into account everything you do to treat your headaches, how well do you think you control them? (please tick one box) | ☐ not at all    ☐ a little    ☐ quite well    ☐ completely |
|---|---|---|

The next questions are about **lost time** because of your headaches.

| 58 | On how many days **in the last 3 months** could you not go to work or school because of your headaches? (please enter the number of days missed completely) | _______ |
|---|---|---|

| 59 | On how many days **in the last 3 months** could you do **less than half** your usual amount in your job or schoolwork because of your headaches? (please enter the number of days; do **not** include days you counted in question 58 where you missed work or school) | _______ |
|---|---|---|

| 60 | On how many days **in the last 3 months** could you not do any household work because of your headaches? (please enter the number of days lost completely) | _______ |
|---|---|---|

| 61 | On how many days **in the last 3 months** could you do **less than half** your usual amount of household work because of your headaches? (please enter the number of days; do **not** include days you counted in question 60 where you did not do any household work) | _______ |
|---|---|---|

| 62 | On how many days **in the last 3 months** did you miss family, social or leisure activities because of your headaches? (please enter the number of days) | _______ |
|---|---|---|

The next questions aim to understand how much your headaches affect you **even when you do not actually have an attack**.

Please think carefully about the last day when you did **not** have a headache (not counting today).

| | | |
|---|---|---|
| **63** | When was the last day when you did **not** have a headache? (please enter the number of days or weeks since your last day **without** headache, or tick the box and go directly to question 67) (if you had **no headache yesterday**, enter 1 day) | ☐ ______ ______ **days**   **weeks**   **cannot remember** |
| **64** | **On that day**, were you anxious or worried about your next headache episode? (please tick one box) | **no** ☐   **yes** ☐ |
| **65** | **On that day**, was there anything you could not do or did not do because you wanted to avoid getting a headache? (please tick one box) | **no** ☐   **yes** ☐ |
| **66** | **On that day**, did you feel **completely free** from all headache-related symptoms? (please tick one box) | **no** ☐   **yes** ☐ |

The next questions ask about **willingness to pay for treatment**.

Imagine that there is a treatment you can buy. If you take it, your headaches will no longer bother you. How much would you be willing to pay **every month** for this treatment?

[These questions are not appropriate in all cultures, and may not be appropriate in countries with free or reimbursed health care. If used, they should apply national currency units (NCU). The multiplier X should be such that reasonable expectation of average willingness to pay is matched by NCU 10X.]

| | | |
|---|---|---|
| **67** | Would you pay NCU 5X a month? (tick one box) If the answer is no, go to question 68; if the answer is yes, go to question 71. | **no** ☐   **yes** ☐ |
| **68** | Would you pay NCU 2X a month? (tick one box) If the answer is no, go to question 69; if the answer is yes, agree an amount between NCU 2X and 5X and go directly to question 75. | **no** ☐   **yes** ☐  **agreed amount: NCU ______** |

| 69 | **Would you pay NCU 1X a month?**<br>(tick one box)<br><br>If the answer is no, go to question 70; if the answer is yes, agree an amount between NCU 1X and 2X and go directly to question 75. | no ☐        yes ☐<br><br>**agreed amount: NCU ______** |
|---|---|---|
| 70 | **Would you pay anything?**<br>(tick one box)<br><br>If the answer is no, go directly to question 75; if the answer is yes, agree an amount between NCU 0 and 1X and go directly to question 75. | no ☐        yes ☐<br><br>**agreed amount: NCU ______** |
| 71 | **Would you pay NCU 10X a month?**<br>(tick one box)<br><br>If the answer is yes, go to question 72; if the answer is no, agree an amount between NCU 5X and 10X and go directly to question 75. | no ☐        yes ☐<br><br>**agreed amount: NCU ______** |
| 72 | **Would you pay NCU 20X a month?**<br>(tick one box)<br><br>If the answer is yes, go to question 73; if the answer is no, agree an amount between NCU 10X and 20X and go directly to question 75. | no ☐        yes ☐<br><br>**agreed amount: NCU ______** |
| 73 | **Would you pay NCU 50X a month?**<br>(tick one box)<br><br>If the answer is yes, go to question 74; if the answer is no, agree an amount between NCU 20X and 50X and go directly to question 74 | no ☐        yes ☐<br><br>**agreed amount: NCU ______** |
| 74 | **Would you pay NCU 100X a month?**<br>(tick one box)<br><br>If the answer is no, agree an amount between NCU 50X and 100X; if the answer is yes, agree an amount of NCU 100X or more. | no ☐        yes ☐<br><br>**agreed amount: NCU ______** |

The next three questions are about the effects your headaches have on your relationships, your love life and your choices in family planning.

Please answer no to any that do not apply.

| 75 | In **the last 3 months**, have your headaches caused difficulties in your love life?<br>(please tick one box) | no ☐        yes ☐ |
|---|---|---|
| 76 | Have your headaches ever caused a long-term relationship or partnership to break down?<br>(please tick one box) | ☐            ☐            ☐<br>no        yes,        yes,<br>temporarily  permanently |

| 77 | Have your headaches affected **your choices** with regard to **family planning**? (please tick all boxes that apply **because of your headaches**) | no ☐<br><br>yes, I have had fewer children ☐<br><br>yes, I have avoided having children ☐<br><br>yes, they have made it harder to conceive ☐<br><br>yes, I have avoided oral contraception ☐ |
|---|---|---|

The next two questions are for **people with children of school age**.

If they do not apply, please go directly to question 80.

| 78 | During **the last 3 months**, have **your** headaches caused one or more of your children to miss school? (please tick one box and, if yes, estimate the total number of missed days) | no ☐   yes ☐<br><br>**total number of days** _______ |
|---|---|---|
| 79 | During **the last 3 months**, have **your** headaches prevented you from taking an interest in your children? (please tick one box) | ☐ **less than once a month**   ☐ **yes, once or more a month**   ☐ **yes, once or more a week**   ☐ **yes, every day** |

The next two sets of questions are for **people with household partners**.

(A household partner may be husband or wife, or an unmarried partner of either gender in a stable relationship.)

If you are not now living with a partner, please go directly to question 87.

| 80 | During **the last 3 months**, have **your** headaches caused **your partner** to lose time from work? (please tick one box and, if yes, enter the total number of days lost) | no ☐   yes ☐<br><br>**total number of days** ____ |
|---|---|---|
| 81 | During **the last 3 months**, have **your** headaches caused **your partner** to miss social activities? (please tick one box and, if yes, enter the total number of occasions missed) | no ☐   yes ☐<br><br>**number of occasions** ____ |

The next five questions are about **your household partner**. We would like to know if your partner has headaches and, if so, how they affect **your** life.

If you are **not** now living with a partner, please go directly to question 87.

| | | |
|---|---|---|
| **82** | Has **your partner** had a headache in the last year?<br>(please tick one box) | no ☐  yes ☐<br>(if no, go directly to question 87) |
| **83** | During **the last 30 days**, on how many days did he/she have a headache?<br>(enter the number of days between 0 and 30) | _______ days |
| **84** | During **the last 3 months**, have **your partner's** headaches caused **you** to lose time from work?<br>(please tick one box and, if yes, enter the total number of days lost) | no ☐  yes ☐<br><br>**total number of days** _____ |
| **85** | During **the last 3 months**, have **your partner's** headaches caused **you** to miss social activities?<br>(please tick one box and, if yes, enter the total number of occasions missed) | no ☐  yes ☐<br><br>**number of occasions** _____ |
| **86** | During **the last 3 months**, have **your partner's** headaches caused difficulties in your love life?<br>(please tick one box) | no ☐  yes ☐ |

The next three series of questions are general, to be **answered by everyone**, with or without headaches.

**Body mass index questions**

Your answers to these questions will give an indication of your level of fitness.

| | | |
|---|---|---|
| **87** | What is your weight?<br>(please enter your weight in kilograms **or** stones and pounds) | _______ kg    _______ st _____ lb |
| **88** | What is your height?<br>(please enter your height in centimetres **or** feet and inches) | _______ cm    _______ ft _____ in |
| **89** | What is your waist measurement?<br>(please measure at the level of the umbilicus (navel) and enter the measurement in centimetres **or** inches)<br><br>Tick the box if you are pregnant. | _______ cm    ☐<br>_______ in    **pregnant** |

## Quality of life questions (WHOQoL-8)

This set of eight questions, developed by the World Health Organization, are for everybody, whether they have headaches or not. They will help us compare people with headaches and people without.

The questions ask how you feel about your quality of life, health or other areas of your life. Each question has five response options. **Please choose the answer that appears most appropriate by circling the number in the appropriate column.** If you are unsure about which response to give to a question, the first response you think of is often the best one.

Please keep in mind your standards, hopes, pleasures and concerns. We ask that you think about your life **in the last 4 weeks.**

| | | very poor | poor | neither poor nor good | good | very good |
|---|---|---|---|---|---|---|
| **90** | How would you rate your quality of life? | 1 | 2 | 3 | 4 | 5 |

| | | very dissatisfied | dissatisfied | neither satisfied nor dissatisfied | satisfied | very satisfied |
|---|---|---|---|---|---|---|
| **91** | How satisfied are you with your health? | 1 | 2 | 3 | 4 | 5 |
| **92** | How satisfied are you with your ability to perform your daily living activities? | 1 | 2 | 3 | 4 | 5 |
| **93** | How satisfied are you with yourself? | 1 | 2 | 3 | 4 | 5 |
| **94** | How satisfied are you with your personal relationships? | 1 | 2 | 3 | 4 | 5 |
| **95** | How satisfied are you with the conditions of your living place? | 1 | 2 | 3 | 4 | 5 |

| | | not at all | a little | moderately | mostly | completely |
|---|---|---|---|---|---|---|
| **96** | Do you have enough energy for everyday life? | 1 | 2 | 3 | 4 | 5 |
| **97** | Have you enough money to meet your needs? | 1 | 2 | 3 | 4 | 5 |

**Subjective wellbeing questions**

These four questions ask how you feel about aspects of your life. Please answer each one on a scale of 0-10, where 0 is "not at all" and 10 is "completely".

| 98 | Overall, how satisfied are you with your life nowadays? (please enter your answer as a number between 0 and 10 where 0 is not at all satisfied and 10 is completely satisfied) | ___________ (enter 0-10) |
|---|---|---|
| 99 | Overall, to what extent do you feel that the things you do in your life are worthwhile? (please enter your answer as a number between 0 and 10 where 0 is not at all worthwhile and 10 is completely worthwhile) | ___________ (enter 0-10) |
| 100 | Overall, how happy did you feel yesterday? (please enter your answer as a number between 0 and 10 where 0 is not at all happy and 10 is completely happy) | ___________ (enter 0-10) |
| 101 | Overall, how anxious did you feel yesterday? (please enter your answer as a number between 0 and 10 where 0 is not at all anxious and 10 is completely anxious) | ___________ (enter 0-10) |

**The questionnaire is now complete. Thank you very much for your time.**

**This section is only for respondents in the validation sub-sample.**

| 201 | Physician-diagnosis of most bothersome headache (if made) | ___________ |
|---|---|---|
| 202 | Physician-diagnosis of other headache 1 (if made) | ___________ |
| 203 | Physician-diagnosis of other headache 2 (if made) | ___________ |
| 204 | Physician-diagnosis of other headache 3 (if made) | ___________ |

Andrée C, Vaillant M, Barré J, Katsarava Z, Lainez JM, Lair ML, et al. Development and validation of the EUROLIGHT questionnaire to evaluate the burden of primary headache disorders in Europe. *Cephalalgia* 2010, 30: 1082–1100. 10.1177/0333102409354323

# Cluster Headache Impact Questionnaire (CHIQ)

**Cluster Headache Impact Questionnaire (CHIQ)**

The aim of this questionnaire is to describe the **CURRENT** impact of cluster headache on your daily life. **Please tick the answer to each question that best describes your condition LAST WEEK.**

1. How often did your headaches have an impact on your ability to work, do housework or meet other responsibilities?

☐ Never        ☐ Rarely        ☐ Sometimes        ☐ Often        ☐ Very often        ☐ Always

2. How often did your headaches have an impact on your family life, leisure activities or social contacts?

☐ Never        ☐ Rarely        ☐ Sometimes        ☐ Often        ☐ Very often        ☐ Always

3. How often have you felt too tired to work or carry out your daily activities because of headaches at night?

☐ Never        ☐ Rarely        ☐ Sometimes        ☐ Often        ☐ Very often        ☐ Always

4. How often were you irritated or fed up with everything because of headaches?

☐ Never        ☐ Rarely        ☐ Sometimes        ☐ Often        ☐ Very often        ☐ Always

5. How often were you afraid to plan anything because of the unpredictability of the headache attacks?

☐ Never        ☐ Rarely        ☐ Sometimes        ☐ Often        ☐ Very often        ☐ Always

6. How often were you unable to think clearly or concentrate even between the attacks?

☐ Never        ☐ Rarely        ☐ Sometimes        ☐ Often        ☐ Very often        ☐ Always

7. How often did you do harmful things to yourself (such as hitting your head or biting the inside of your cheek) when you had a headache?

☐ Never        ☐ Rarely        ☐ Sometimes        ☐ Often        ☐ Very often        ☐ Always

8. How often did you feel you were a burden to others because of your headaches?

☐ Never        ☐ Rarely        ☐ Sometimes        ☐ Often        ☐ Very often        ☐ Always

How many attacks did you have altogether last week? _____ attacks

How often did you take acute medication for your cluster headaches last week? _____ triptans/oxygen

Kamm, K., Straube, A. & Ruscheweyh, R. Cluster Headache Impact Questionnaire (CHIQ) – a short measure of cluster headache related disability. *J Headache Pain* **23**, 37 (2022). https://doi.org/10.1186/s10194-022-01406-y

# Headache Disability Questionnaire (HDQ)

**HEADACHE DISABILITY INDEX QUESTIONNAIRE**

*Documentation*

LAST NAME: _______________________ FIRST NAME: ________________ MI: ____ Date: __________________

Please CHECK the correct response:

I have headaches:  ○ 1 per month  ○ more than 1 but less than 4 per month      ○ more than 1 per week

My headache is:  ○ Mild      ○ Moderate      ○ Severe

| | | YES | SOMETIMES | NO |
|---|---|---|---|---|
| E1 | Because of my headaches I feel handicapped. | ○ | ○ | ○ |
| F2 | Because of my headaches I feel restricted in performing my routine daily activities. | ○ | ○ | ○ |
| E3 | No one understands the effect my headaches have on my life. | ○ | ○ | ○ |
| F4 | I restrict my recreational activities (e.g. sports, hobbies) because of my headaches. | ○ | ○ | ○ |
| E5 | My headaches make me angry. | ○ | ○ | ○ |
| E6 | Sometimes I feel that I am going to lose control because of my headaches. | ○ | ○ | ○ |
| F7 | Because of my headaches I am less likely to socialize. | ○ | ○ | ○ |
| E8 | My spouse (significant other), or family and friends have no idea what I am going through because of my headaches. | ○ | ○ | ○ |
| E9 | My headaches are so bad that I feel that I am going to go insane. | ○ | ○ | ○ |
| E10 | My outlook on the world is affected by my headaches. | ○ | ○ | ○ |
| E11 | I am afraid to go outside when I feel that a headache is starting. | ○ | ○ | ○ |
| E12 | I feel desperate because of my headaches. | ○ | ○ | ○ |
| F13 | I am concerned that I am paying penalties at work or at home because of my headaches. | ○ | ○ | ○ |
| E14 | My headaches place stress on my relationships with family or friends. | ○ | ○ | ○ |
| F15 | I avoid being around people when I have a headache. | ○ | ○ | ○ |
| F16 | I believe my headaches are making it difficult for me to achieve my goals in life. | ○ | ○ | ○ |
| F17 | I am unable to think clearly because of my headaches. | ○ | ○ | ○ |
| F18 | I get tense (e.g. muscle tension) because of my headaches. | ○ | ○ | ○ |
| F19 | I do not enjoy social gatherings because of my headaches. | ○ | ○ | ○ |
| E20 | I feel irritable because of my headaches. | ○ | ○ | ○ |
| F21 | I avoid traveling because of my headaches. | ○ | ○ | ○ |
| E22 | My headaches make me feel confused. | ○ | ○ | ○ |
| E23 | My headaches make me feel frustrated | ○ | ○ | ○ |
| F24 | I find it difficult to read because of my headaches. | ○ | ○ | ○ |
| F25 | I find it difficult to focus my attention away from my headaches and on other things. | ○ | ○ | ○ |

K Niere, M Quin. Development of a headache-specific disability questionnaire for patients attending physiotherapy. Man Ther, 2009; 14:45-51. DOI: https://doi.org/10.1016/j.math.2007.09.006